Dedication

I dedicate this book to Pepi, my w
cannot give you enough th
and thoroughly ha

This book is also
grandchild, born March
Your big sister Isabel will

I would like to thank the fol
Publishers, David Cella, Lisa Go
their help and guidance.

Guide for the New Health Care Professional

Ron Scott, EdD, JD, LLM, PT
Attorney-Mediator and Clinical Physical Therapist
San Antonio, Texas

1610

JONES AND BARTLETT PUBLISHERS
Sudbury, Massachusetts
BOSTON   TORONTO   LONDON   SINGAPORE

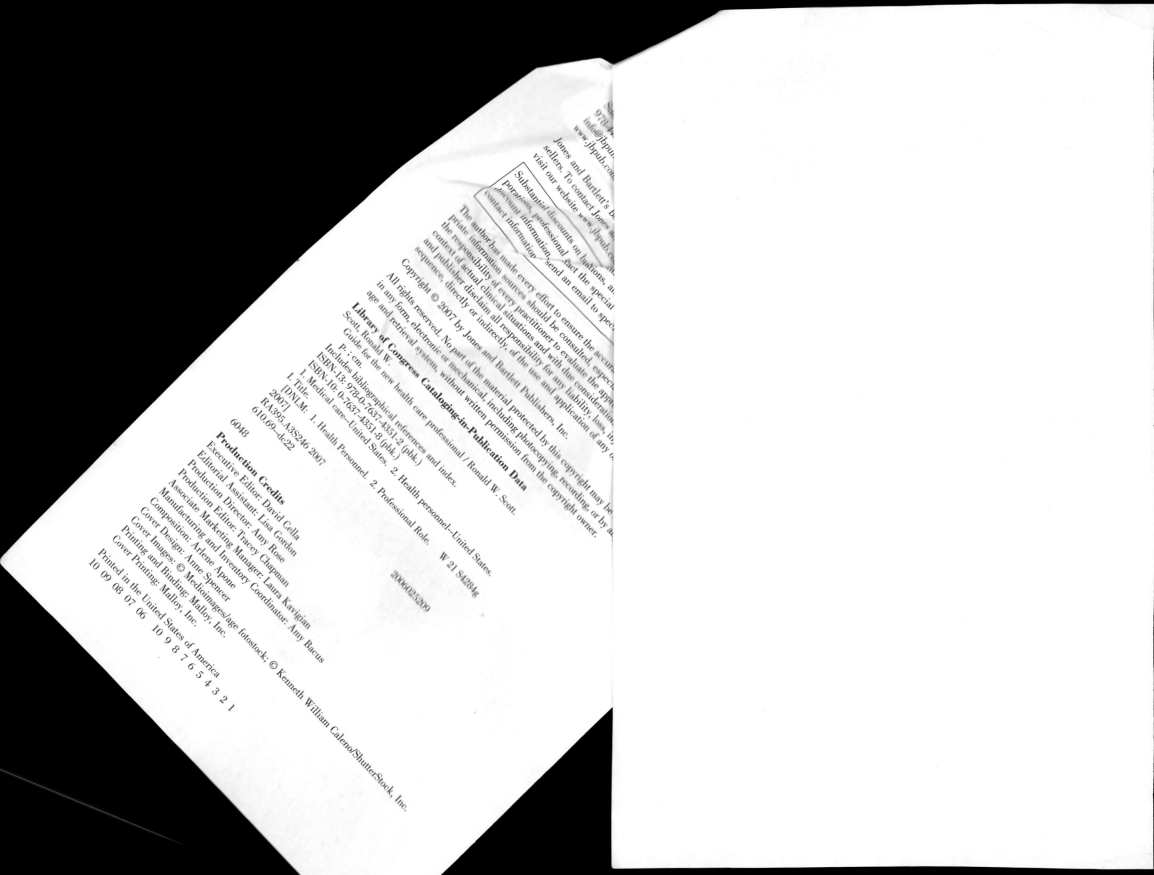

Su...
978-...
info@jbpub...
www.jbpub.co...
Jones and Bartlett's b...
sellers. To contact Jones a...
visit our website www.jbpub.co...

Substantial discounts on bulk quantities, a...
porations, professional, professional fact the special...
discount information send an email to spec...
contact information

Library of Congress Cataloging-in-Publication Data

Scott, Ronald W.
    Guide for the new health care professional / Ronald W. Scott.
        p. ; cm.
    Includes bibliographical references and index.
    ISBN-13: 978-0-7637-4351-2 (pbk.)
    ISBN-10: 0-7637-4351-8 (pbk.)
    1. Title.
    [DNLM: 1. Health Personnel. 2. Professional Role.   W 21 S42846
2007]
    RA395.A3S246 2007
    610.69—dc22
                                                                    2006025209

6048

Production Credits
Executive Editor: David Cella
Editorial Assistant: Lisa Gordon
Production Director: Amy Rose
Production Editor: Tracey Chapman
Associate Marketing Manager: Laura Kavigian
Manufacturing and Inventory Coordinator: Amy Bacus
Composition: Arlene Apone
Cover Design: Anne Spencer
Cover Images: © Medioimages/age fotostock; © Kenneth William Caleno/ShutterStock, Inc.
Printing and Binding: Malloy, Inc.
Cover Printing: Malloy, Inc.

Printed in the United States of America
10 09 08 07 06   10 9 8 7 6 5 4 3 2 1

About the Author

Ron Scott, EdD, JD, LLM, PT, is a practicing attorney, educator, and health care professional, dividing his work time among the three disciplines. Ron began his health care career as a Navy hospital corpsman and operating room technician in 1970. He left military service initially in 1973 to study physical therapy at the University of Pittsburgh. Ron has been a clinical physical therapist since 1977.

Ron attended law school at the University of San Diego from 1980 to 1983, where he was law review editor and symposium editor for the school's prestigious *Law of the Sea* issue. He subsequently served as an Army attorney–prosecutor and chief of international law in Frankfurt, Germany. After his return to the United States, Ron earned his postdoctoral Master of Laws (LLM) degree from the Judge Advocate General's School in Charlottesville, Virginia. He then worked as an Army medical claims judge advocate until 1989.

Ron finished his 20-year military career as a physical therapy clinic director and senior staff member at Fort Polk, Louisiana and Fort Sam Houston, Texas. He retired from the Army in 1994 as a Major in the Medical Specialist Corps.

From 1994 to 1998, Ron was a member of the faculty, and from 1995 to 1996, he was acting chair of the Physical Therapy Department at the University of Texas Health Science Center at San Antonio. He has been adjunct faculty and/or lecturer in a number of graduate health education programs since 1996, including Hahnemann University, Husson College, Lebanon Valley College, Marymount University, Northern Arizona University, Rocky Mountain University, University of Indianapolis, and Webster University.

Ron has published nine books, most recently *Legal Aspects of Documenting Patient Care for Rehabilitation Professionals,* 3rd edition, Jones and Bartlett (2006). Ron has also published over 60 articles on topics ranging from cleidocranial dysplasia to health law and ethics to protecting U.S. interests in Antarctica.

Ron's current legal interests focus on mediation of interpersonal disputes.

Contents

Preface

An editorial in the Sunday *London Times* declared on November 3, 2002, that health care human resource management is as important as life and death, and as critical to successful patient care outcomes as is the clinical delivery of health care services itself. The inference to be drawn from this bold assertion is that it is the work of health care professionals in multiple supporting roles that makes health care service delivery successful. You currently are contemplating becoming, or are about to become, such a professional. Welcome to one of the most exciting and rewarding work environments on Earth!

This book describes in detail the requisites and traits of the consummate health care professional. The book begins by exploring the health care milieu and its component parts—patients and their significant others, professionals, disciplines, organizations, systems, payers, and governments. The nature of the health care interdisciplinary team is explored with the theme of patient-centered care. The concept of "professionalism" is examined from its historic roots to present day. Morals, ethics, and legal duties are defined and distinguished. Core professional attributes and values are discussed through real-life and hypothetical case examples. Select health care legal and ethical duties are presented and exemplified. Job search strategies and tactics are discussed, including exemplars of resumes and cover letters. Tactics and strategies for professional and personal growth and job retention are explored. Areas of potential interpersonal disputes and conflict development, intervention, and resolution are examined. The book ends with a discussion of career changes, with personal inventories for readers to use in examining their own career paths.

Each chapter begins with an abstract and a list of key words and objectives, presents relevant chapter exercises, and ends with a series of questions and/or cases for thought and a list of references, readings, and resources. Hypothetical cases drawn from real-life experiences are dispersed throughout the book.

Best wishes for practice success!

Chapter 1

Individuals and Teams in Health Care Service Delivery

ABSTRACT

Health care professionals—as individuals and as members of teams—are vital to successful patient outcomes. Teams may be multidisciplinary, such as complementary medical group practices operating out of the same outpatient setting. Interdisciplinary teams work in concert throughout patients' course of care, such as surgical and rehabilitation teams. The five domains of health professional clinical practice include the following: examination, evaluation, diagnosis, prognosis, and intervention on patients' behalf. Just as health care professionals have formidable responsibilities, so do patients in support of their own recovery. These patient duties are memorialized in patient bills of rights and responsibilities.

KEY WORDS AND PHRASES

- Advanced practice nurse
- Allied health
- Cerebrovascular accident
- Contract for (health) services
- Doctor of Medicine
- Doctor of Osteopathic Medicine
- Dysfunction
- Express contractual duty
- Etiology
- Home health agency
- Implied contractual duty
- Interdisciplinary team
- Licensed practical nurse
- Managed care
- Multidisciplinary team
- Nurse anesthetist
- Nurse midwife
- Nurse practitioner

- Patient Bill of Rights and Responsibilities
- Physical therapist
- *Pro bono* services
- Prosthetist
- Occupational therapist
- Optimal therapeutic outcome
- Orthotist
- Registered nurse

- Rehabilitation team
- Situational leadership
- Social worker
- Speech–language pathologist
- Surgical team
- Therapeutic contract
- Third-party reimbursement
- Work-around
- Work–life balance

OBJECTIVES

1. Distinguish multidisciplinary and interdisciplinary health care teams.
2. Compare the roles and patient care responsibilities of select key health care professionals.
3. Analyze leadership in health care clinical service delivery.
4. Evaluate the need for "work–life" balance for every professional.
5. Recognize patient responsibilities for successful health care outcomes.
6. Delineate the patient and health professional's legal contractual duties incident to the therapeutic contract for care.

"No man or woman is an island." "It takes a village." "I am an Army of one." "A team is only as strong as its weakest link." The first two common phrases are seemingly in conflict with the latter two. How can a team and an individual simultaneously be equally important?

In health care, they are equally important. The interdisciplinary team of professionals caring for patients and clients acts a lot like an orchestra, often, but not always, led by a physician "conductor." Its work in concert supports and very often saves patients' lives. Each individual on the team also supports and saves lives through his or her individual work effort. It does take a "village" of health care professionals, in many roles and at many levels, working together to make patient care highly successful; however, no team can work without everyone on board functioning at his or her best. Individuals make the health care team what it is.

> Individual health care professionals at all levels work individually and in concert with others to make health care teams successful!

Multidisciplinary and Interdisciplinary Health Care Professional Teams

In any profession, but particularly in clinical health care delivery, knowledge of team dynamics is important. According to Grumbach and Bodenheimer, health care teams have five basic characteristics: clear goals with measurable outcomes, clinical and administrative system structures, pre-established division of work effort, systematic training of all team members in vital team processes, and effective communication.

How health care teams interact determines whether patients live or die. At a less emergent level, effective, cohesive teams facilitate improved patient outcomes of care and satisfaction with the care received. Health care teams are of two basic types—multidisciplinary and interdisciplinary.

Multidisciplinary teams include health professionals from complementary or disparate health care disciplines co-located in the same site. They may support each other—even refer patients to each other; however, they generally care for their patients in a compartmentalized fashion, without a shared conceptual framework. An example of a multidisciplinary team includes the tenants in an outpatient health center, composed of orthopedists, radiologists, occupational, physical and speech therapists, and clinical psychologists.

Interdisciplinary teams, such as hospital-based surgical and rehabilitation teams, work closely together from the commencement of patient care through discharge of patients in pursuit of shared goals. Interdisciplinary health professional teams are generally headed by a physician team leader.

In surgery, team members work seamlessly to carry out required and elective operations on patients. Surgical team members include surgeons, anesthesiologists and/or nurse anesthetists, registered and licensed practical nurses (registered nurses [RNs] and licensed practical nurses [LPNs]), surgical technologists (formerly operating room technicians), radiology technicians (x-ray technicians), medical photographers, and relevant others.

In rehabilitation, health professional team members share time during the treatment day with patients, alternating or simultaneously providing care. They meet together regularly and on an *ad hoc* basis for team conferences about the patients under their care. Rehabilitation patients include, among others, cardiac rehabilitation patients, patients with spinal cord injuries, postoperative orthopedic patients, and stroke patients.

Being a team leader is not necessarily easy, although it is highly necessary and rewarding. A leader must be able to compel others to do what they might not otherwise do in order to accomplish the team's mission related to patient care. Under Blanchard's situational leadership model, a leader may, depending on circumstances, be highly directive and supportive (microman-ager), provide subordinates with low direction and support (delegator), or provide direction and support somewhere in between. According to Rooke and Torbert, leaders are made, not born, and how they develop is critical to mission and organizational success. Brounstein noted that leaders must manage three primary areas in team management: responsibility, account-ability, and conflict management.

Fandray pointed out that a leader must know the team and organization from top to bottom and everywhere in between. He or she must be ready and willing to get hands dirty and to get all things done through his or her people resources, without interfering unduly in their work. According to Brousseau, leaders must

> The main goal of health professional interven-tion is to facilitate optimal patient thera-peutic outcomes.

be decisive and flexible, taking maximal advan-tage of information presented to them. Although high-level leaders are "strategists" who set an organization and teams' missions, front-line leaders and their staffs are the "tacticians" who give the organization's mission effect—that is, they make it happen!

Profiles of Select Health Care Professionals

The following descriptive list of health professionals is not intended to be all-inclusive, but rather representative of the myriad of primary and support pro-fessionals who carry out patient care.

Doctors

Physicians and surgeons serve a fundamental role in our society and have an important effect on all of our lives. As primary (first-order, independent) health care providers, they carry out the five main parameters of primary health care practice. They examine patients and obtain medical histories; order, per-form, and interpret diagnostic tests; make relevant evaluative findings from their examinations, tests, and measurements;

> The five parameters of primary health profes-sional clinical practice include: examination, evaluation, diagnosis, prognosis and interven-tion on patients' behalf.

diagnose and formulate prognoses (predic-tions about the course of diseases and patients' recovery); and intervene on patients' behalf. They also counsel patients on diet, hygiene, and preventive health care. Surgeons perform oper-ations on patients and specialize by body sys-tems, from cardiopulmonary to gynecologic and obstetric to neurologic to urologic surgery.

There are two types of physicians: MD—Doctor of Medicine—and DO— Doctor of Osteopathic Medicine. MDs are also known as allopathic physicians. Although both MDs and DOs may use all accepted methods of treatment, including drugs and surgery, DOs place special emphasis on the body's musculoskeletal system, preventive medicine, and holistic patient care. DOs are more likely than MDs to be primary care specialists, although they can be found in all specialties. About half of DOs practice general or family medicine, internal medicine, or pediatrics.

Many physicians—primarily general and family practitioners, internists, pediatricians, obstetricians and gynecologists, and psychiatrists—work in small, private offices or clinics, often assisted by a small staff of nurses and other administrative personnel. Increasingly, physicians, like most other health care professionals, practice within health care organizations, thus providing backup coverage and allowing for more individual time off, facilitating an improved individual work–life balance.

Work–life balance—balancing divided loyalties to and sharing finite time among employers, patients and clients, family, friends and oneself—is critically important to the personal well-being of health care professionals. Although there are many tactics and strategies offered to improve and achieve work–life balance, the fundamental ones must include simplifying one's personal life, managing individual and collective stress, minimizing "work-arounds" (redundancies) in the workplace, expending equitable energy and time on all high-priority agendas in one's life, and alternating work activities to avoid burnout.

A recent survey by the Doctors Company (the largest physician-owned medical liability company) found that fewer physicians are encouraging their children to become physicians. Reasons cited for this trend include the threat of litigation, job stress, and fewer tangible rewards from the practice of medicine.

On a more positive note, in a recent article about the complex world and work of neurosurgeons—medical specialists who operate on central nervous system organs—Grimes described a book by neurosurgeon Katrina Firlik, *Another Day in the Frontal Lobe: A Brain Surgeon Exposes Life on the Inside* (Random House, 2006). Here Dr. Firlik characterizes neurosurgeons as a combination of scientist, mechanic, manual laborer, and computer specialist. Precision and dedication are two of the main hallmarks of any health professional.

Nurses

Nurses make up the largest block of health care professionals, with over 2.4 million registered and licensed practical and vocational nurses in active practice. Nurses staff three of five hospital positions. As the most global care providers with the most variegated range of disparate professional roles, nurses epitomize the image of *the* health care professional. A November 2005

Gallup poll of consumers reported that people trust nurses more than they do any other class of professionals.

RNs provide high-level care for patients across the spectrum of age, gender, and pathologies. They take patient histories and make and record nursing assessments on patients, carry out complex patient treatments, administer medications in all modes of delivery, operate complex medical machinery, and carry out patient and family education on an ongoing basis. RNs also support physicians in carrying out and interpreting diagnostic tests and measurements on their patients.

RNs interact on an ongoing basis with all other health care professionals and are the gatekeepers for access to patients by all relevant others. RNs in clinical practice also interact regularly with patients' families and significant others and teach them and their patients home- and self-care procedures. They carry out grief counseling for families of patients at one end of the life spectrum and preventive health screening at the other for patients and clients from all walks of life.

RNs often specialize at the basic nursing level by work setting or by patient condition, age, or gender. A sample of nurse specialties includes ambulatory care nurses, critical care and trauma nurses, geriatric nurses, neonatal nurses, occupational health nurses, psychiatric nurses, surgical nurses, and transplant nurses.

RNs may also specialize through postprofessional study and practice to become advanced practice nurses. These specialties include nurse practitioners, who may practice independently; nurse midwives, who deliver babies; and nurse anesthetists, who administer anesthesia to patients undergoing surgical procedures.

RNs enter the field via either associate or bachelor's degree programs or through approved certificates programs. They work in a wide variety of settings, from hospitals and hospices to outpatient facilities and schools to home health agencies to professional education and research settings.

There is an ongoing severe shortage of registered nurses in the United States. According to the U.S. Department of Health and Human Services, by 2020, demand for RNs in the United States will exceed supply by 800,000. The shortage issue is exacerbated by the fact that the median age for RNs is rising and many RNs are leaving the field through attrition or retirement or are choosing part-time

---

Duties of registered nurses include the following:

- Patient assessment (initial, ongoing, and at discharge)
- Patient histories
- Medication administration
- Operation of complex medical equipment and machinery
- Patient and family education and counseling
- Preventive health screening
- Treatment

instead of full-time employment. At the same time, as medical technology grows, RNs constitute the second largest growth profession among all professions through 2014.

To ease the shortage of registered nurses, in part, by hospitals, health care systems and professional associations are aggressively recruiting foreign-educated nurses. Immigration laws ease their immigration into this country. This draining of vital health professional resources, however, exacts a great toll on the nurses' homelands, some of which are demanding compensation for the exiting professionals' exodus, according to an excellent *New York Times* article by Dugger.

LPNs care for injured and ill patients under the direction of RNs and physicians. As part of their duties, they take patient vital signs (temperature, pulse, respiration rate, and blood pressure). LPNs also apply wound dressings, give injections, help deliver and care for babies, monitor catheters and intravenous lines, and treat bedsores, among other medical procedures. In states where permitted, LPNs also administer medications and commence intravenous therapy.

LPNs may supervise aides, nursing assistants, and LPN students. Approximately 750,000 LPNs are in active practice in the United States. LPN professional preparation involves approximately 1 year of classroom and clinical education. LPNs work in similar settings as RNs. Like RNs (who take the NCLEX-RN), they undertake a state-administered licensing examination to qualify to practice—the NCLEX-PN.

> As part of their official duties, licensed practical and vocational nurses take patient vital signs: temperature, pulse and respiration rate (TPR) and blood pressure (BP) and provide bedside care for patients.

Occupational and Physical Therapists

Occupational therapists (OTs) and physical therapists (PTs) had their genesis from the same profession—"reconstruction aides" recruited by the U.S. military to treat wounded soldiers during World War I. After the war, the two distinct disciplines formed, and each developed a disparate scope of practice. Modernly, the two professions perform the same or similar work and normally work together as complementary professional health care disciplines in multiple rehabilitation settings.

OTs assist patients in optimizing work skills and regaining proficiency in carrying out activities of daily living (ADLs). Their clientele includes patients with physical, mental, and developmental impairments and disabilities.

They use physical exercise regimes to increase patient muscle strength, as needed. OTs use their professional skills to help patients improve abstract

OTs evaluate and care for patients and clients with physical and/or mental disease or injuries. They help to restore patient function for return to work and for optimization of ADLs. They carry out preventive health care activities, including, but not limited to, workplace ergonomic evaluations, work place modifications and job redesign, and fabrication of orthoses for patients. They are primary consultants in school settings for students with special needs.

reasoning, hand–eye and whole body coordination, and memory and perceptual skills. They consult with workers and industry to modify work places and carry out ergonomic evaluations and redesign jobs to fit workers' needs. OTs fabricate, apply, and modify orthoses (splints) to patients under their care.

OTs also work with patients in mental health settings. They help patients develop coping, stress-management, and time-management skills, among other skill sets.

There are nearly 100,000 OTs in active practice. OTs work in virtually every setting where patients and clients are found, especially including school settings. They supervise certified occupational therapy assistants (COTAs) and rehabilitation aides and work closely with physical therapists and speech pathologists.

Entry-level professional education for OTs is currently at the baccalaureate, master's, or doctoral levels, but will be exclusively at the graduate level commencing in 2007. OTs undertake licensing examinations similar to physical therapists in order to qualify for practice. The American Occupational Therapy Association—the professional association for OTs and COTAs—has one of the most comprehensive ethics codes of any health care discipline.

Chapter Exercise 1

Please take a few minutes to access, review, and assess the Occupational Therapy Code of Ethics at www.aota.org.

PTs carry out therapeutic activities similar to OTs, except that their involvement in mental health settings is more limited. PTs work with patients and clients of all ages to restore physical function after injury or illness. They design and carry out exercises for patients, administer simple to complex tests and measurements of patient function, care for patients with burns and wounds, and administer cardiopulmonary interventions, among other therapeutic activities.

PTs make extensive use of assistive and adaptive devices in support of patient recovery, including, but not limited to, canes, crutches, walkers, and wheelchairs of all kinds. They apply manual and mechanical traction to patients with spinal dysfunction and use manual therapy techniques such as mobilization to restore optimal joint function. They use physical modalities such as electrical stimulation and ultrasound heat as adjuncts to hands-on care.

There are approximately 100,000 PTs in active practice. They work closely with physical therapist assistants (PTAs), aides, and other support professionals in their practices. Entry-level professional education is at the master's or doctoral level. Substantial volunteer experience or exposure is a prerequisite to gaining admission to most physical therapy education programs.

> PTs use exercise, manual therapy, and physical modalities to help restore patient function after injury or disease. They are complemented by PTAs in most settings.

Physical therapy may be the only allied health discipline in which the entire scope of practice is spelled out in a comprehensive written practice manual—the *Guide to Physical Therapist Practice.* There are distinct advantages and disadvantages to such a comprehensive practice guide. Such a guide makes the discipline's practice transparent to all concerned—providers, payers, patients, educators, and governmental entities. It also may create a self-imposed legal standard of care that is higher than the law would ordinarily require of practitioners in a discipline.

Speech–Language Pathologists

Speech–language pathologists work with patients and clients with speech, language, swallowing, and cognitive disorders. Such disorders may result from brain injury, cerebral palsy, cleft palate, developmental delay, emotional disorders, or stroke (cerebrovascular accident), among other causes or etiologies.

After evaluating patients, speech–language pathologists use special techniques and devices to improve patients' communicative speaking and writing abilities. Depending on their evaluative findings and patient needs, they may recommend and employ alternative methods of communication, such as sign language or automated devices. They help patients overcome swallowing dysfunction and strengthen relevant muscles for speaking or swallowing. They also work with patients' families and significant others to educate them about impediments to effective communication at home. The overall goal of treatment is to optimize patient function in educational, social, and work settings.

There are approximately 102,000 speech–language pathologists in active practice in the United States. Approximately half of all speech–language pathologists work in school settings, whereas the other half are employed in health care or social services environments. Speech–language pathologists' entry-level education is at the graduate-degree (master's) level. They are required by law to be licensed in most (47 of 50) states if they are employed in health care. Licensure is also a requisite to third-party reimbursement for patient care services. All speech–language pathologists take a national certification examination, and many undertake postprofessional clinical internships as prerequisites to practice. Speech–language pathologists work closely with allied health professionals in clinical settings and with teachers and education administrators in educational settings.

Orthotists and Prosthetists

Orthotists and prosthetists are health professionals who custom design, fabricate, apply, monitor, adjust, and modify braces (orthoses) and artificial limbs (prostheses) for patients. Orthotics and prosthetics (O&P) professionals are mixed product–service professions in that they have dual primary roles as medical product manufacturers and providers of health professional services. O&P professionals simultaneously use routinely high-level cognitive and psychomotor skills in their intensely hands-on work. They work closely with other rehabilitation professionals in interdisciplinary health care settings, including physicians, OTs and PTs, and their assistants and nurses.

There are several distinct classes of professionals within O&P. These include practitioners, assistants, and technicians. O&P practitioners are the lead direct care professionals in O&P. They may be certified in either orthotics or prosthetics or in both.

O&P practitioners undergo the most comprehensive education of the listed professionals and are certified by the American Board for Certification (ABC), which also writes, revises, and enforces the O&P *Cannons of Ethical Conduct* for O&P professionals. There are only eight practitioner professional education programs in the United States, the majority at the postbaccalaureate master's or certificate level. There are approximately 5,000 certified practitioners in active practice in the United States.

Registered assistants work under the supervision of practitioners in certified facilities. Like practitioners, they have a direct patient care role. They adjust, maintain, and repair orthoses and prostheses for patients. As of the time of writing this book, there was only one assistant education program in the United States—Oklahoma State University at Okmulgee. Technicians fabricate and repair orthoses and prostheses according to patient measurements but do not carry out direct patient care.

Social Workers

Social workers are professionals who assist patients and clients in coping with their environments and problems, issues, and dilemmas in their lives. Social problems that social workers confront include, among many others, AIDS, disability, employment, illness, injury, housing, and physical and substance abuse.

Over 90% of social workers are employed in health care and social service agency settings. They interact intensively with their clients.

Most social workers specialize. Areas of specialization include, among others, child, domestic partner, elder, medical, mental health, public health, school, and substance abuse social work. Social workers in physical rehabilitation settings work in concert with physicians, nurses, occupational, physical and speech–language therapists, and others on rehabilitation teams.

More than half a million social workers are in active practice. Their minimum educational credential is the Bachelor of Social Work (BSW) degree. A master's degree in social work (MSW) is typically required for professionals in health care settings and clinical (mental health and substance abuse) social workers. To teach at the university level, professionals in the field typically earn the Doctor of Social Work (DSW) or Doctor of Philosophy (PhD) degree in social work. Depending on the particular state in which the social work professional is employed, certification, licensure, or registration may be required. In a majority of states, licensure—the highest and most intensely scrutinized form of credentialing—requires 2 years (3,000 contact hours) of supervised experience for clinical social workers.

Patient Responsibilities in Treatment

Health care professionals have formidable legal and professional ethical duties that govern their practice and professional interaction with their patients. These responsibilities are discussed in greater detail in Chapters 2 and 3.

Patients and clients also have legal duties incident to care. Every interaction between health care professionals and patients entails legal responsibilities for both or all parties. Even where a formal express business contract for services is not executed, health care professionals and patients each have distinct implied (presumed by law) legal duties.

The basic implied contractual legal duty owed by health care professionals to their patients is to use their best clinical judgment and skills to effect an optimal therapeutic result. Health care professionals are not guarantors of specific therapeutic results, unless they contract to meet such goals.

> Every health care professional has the legal duty to use her or his best clinical judgment and skills to effect an optimal therapeutic result for patients and clients under care.

Managed care—the current health care delivery model—may make it more difficult to meet this implied legal responsibility. With its primary focus on cost-containment, managed care causes health care professionals and organizations to cut costs associated with care delivery to the minimum required to meet the legal standard of care. As a result, a less-than-optimal therapeutic result of care may result for patients.

Despite the problems facing it, the health care delivery system has a lot to be proud of. In a recent article, Arbuckle cited improved patient outcomes from research, reduction of medical errors in the California medical system, innovative human resources management strategies to recruit and retain scarce health care professionals, and partnerships with businesses to increase patient services and community outreach as examples of the good things being accomplished by the health care system.

Patients as well as their health care providers have express and implied legal contractual duties incident to health care delivery. Unless health care services are provided *pro bono* (without cost), patients have the express or implied duty to pay the reasonable value for those services. Most of the time, patients execute this obligation through third-party payers or insurers. Patients also can and should be asked by their providers to promise to help jointly establish and take responsibility for complying with established patient care goals to the maximum extent possible.

Health care organizations and systems have established patient bills of rights and responsibilities, modeled after the original document published by the American Hospital Association. Such a declaration serves to apprise patients and their significant others not only of what they are entitled to from the health care delivery system, but also what is expected of patients in the process. Patient bills of rights and responsibilities are normally prominently posted in patient admission and clinic reception areas, in English, Spanish, and other languages, as needed for effective provider–patient communication.

> Health care professionals are not guarantors of specific therapeutic results.

Copies of the Patient Rights and Responsibilities documents for Brooke Army Medical Center (BAMC), San Antonio, Texas, appear in Appendix A and Appendix B in English and Spanish. I am very grateful to BAMC for the use of its Patient Rights and Responsibilities documents and for its superlative, compassionate professional care for active duty military service members injured in Iraq and Afghanistan. Kudos!

Chapter Exercise 2

Access the Bureau of Labor Statistics website at www.bls.gov and research the professional roles, educational requirements, work settings, salary/wage ranges, and other information of interest for the following principal assistants to primary health care professionals described in this chapter:

- Certified occupational therapy assistant
- Licensed practical nurse
- Physical therapist assistant
- Physician assistant
- Registered orthotic and prosthetic assistant

QUESTIONS AND CASES FOR STUDY

1. Leadership operates along a continuum, where leadership styles may change depending on contingencies. Under which circumstances might strong, centralized micromanagement be necessary? When is a more relaxed, decentralized leadership/management style appropriate, in which subordinates exercise maximum professional autonomy and judgment?

2. Identify steps that professionals in your discipline, and you personally, can undertake to minimize negative stressors that may adversely affect your lives and well-being.

3. What steps can and should governments at multiple levels and private industry undertake to increase the numbers of nurses in active professional practice and to facilitate their remaining in active practice?

4. Consider the "turf wars" over scope of practice and jurisdiction that affect select health care disciplines. What strategies and tactics can be employed—within and without the affected professions—to minimize the occurrence of such potentially destructive phenomena? Who is harmed by such practice wars?

5. Identify discipline-specific patient responsibilities and rights that should be incorporated into a patient bill of responsibilities and rights.

REFERENCES, READINGS, AND RESOURCES

1. Arbuckle B. A lot to cheer about, too: Much lamented medical system also can work miracles. *San Francisco Chronicle.* May 1, 2005, C3.

2. Bassett J. Legal action: APTA files suit against federation of state boards of PT. *Advance for Physical Therapists and PT Assistants.* Dec. 6, 2004, 11.

3. Blanchard K, Zigarmi C, Zigarmi D. *Leadership and the One-Minute Manager.* New York: Blanchard Management Corporation, 1985.

4. Boyle D. Life Etc. What's always worked: Registered nurse. *AARP.* May/June 2006, 88.

5. Brousseau KR. The seasoned executive's decision making style. *Harvard Business Review.* Feb. 2006, 111–120.

6. Dugger CW. Plan to lure nurses to U.S. may harm homelands. *New York Times.* May 24, 2006, A1, 11.

7. Fandray D. Getting things done. *Continental Magazine.* Oct. 2005, 86–88.

8. Firlik K. *Another Day in the Frontal Lobe: A Brain Surgeon Exposes Life on the Inside.* New York: Random House, 2006.

9. Friedman A. Interns' hours shorter, and that's good for patients. *New York Times.* Jan. 24, 2006, D6.

10. Grimes W. Maybe brain surgeons aren't as smart as you think. *New York Times.* May 11, 2006, A33.

11. Grumbach K, Bodenheimer T. Can health care teams improve primary care practice? *Journal of the American Medical Association.* 2004;291:1246–1251.

12. Healing stories. *San Antonio Express News Nurses Week.* May 7, 2006, 4N–5N.

13. Heinemann GD, Zeiss AM (eds.). *Team Performance in Health Care: Assessment and Development.* New York: Springer, 2002.

14. Mallon F. *Memorandum: Draft Report on the Feasibility and Advisability of Direct Access to Physical Therapists.* Alexandria, VA: American Physical Therapy Association, Nov. 4, 2004.

15. *Occupational Outlook Handbook.* Bureau of Labor Statistics, U.S. Department of Labor, 2006.

16. Rooke D, Torbert WR. 7 Transformations of leadership. *Harvard Business Review.* Apr. 2005, 66–76.

17. Scott RW. *Foundations of Physical Therapy.* New York: McGraw-Hill, 2002.

18. Silver S. Are you a fit for critical care nursing? *San Antonio Express News Nurses Week.* May 7, 2006, 2N, 6N.

19. Silverman MJ, Hairston MJ. A descriptive study of private practice in music therapy. *Journal of Music Therapy.* Winter 2005, 262–272.

20. Spear S. Fixing health care from the inside, today. *Harvard Business Review.* Sept. 2005, 78–91.

21. Swindoll Luci. *Notes to a working woman: Finding balance, passion and fulfillment in your life.* Nashville, TN: W. Publishing Group, 2005.

22. *Taber's Cyclopedic Medical Dictionary*, 19th ed. Philadelphia: F.A. Davis, 2001.

23. Top nurses combine skills, compassion. *San Antonio Express News Nurses Week.* May 7, 2006, 3N, 7N.

24. Who will be tomorrow's doctors? Survey finds physicians no longer encouraging their children to become doctors. *Herald: Prime Time Newspapers.* Dec. 29, 2005, 17.

25. Zaroff L. A bout with addition, for the doctor who has everything. *New York Times.* May 9, 2006, D5.

26. www.aha.org (American Hospital Association)

27. www.ama-assn.org (American Medical Association)

28. www.ana.org (American Nurses Association)

29. www.aota.org (American Occupational Therapy Association)

30. www.apta.org (American Physical Therapy Association)

31. www.asha.org (American Speech-Language-Hearing Association)

32. www.napnes.org (National Association for Practical Nurse Education and Service)

33. www.oandp.org (American Academy of Orthotists and Prosthetists)

34. www.socialworkers.org (National Association of Social Workers)

35. www.thedoctors.com (medical liability insurer)

Chapter 2

Professionalism: History, Applications, and Values

ABSTRACT

In the Middle Ages, three basic professions were recognized—the clergy, law and medicine. Its members were part of an exclusive club that controlled education and knowledge itself. As the Industrial Revolution took hold in the 18th and 19th centuries, more and more occupational disciplines legitimately claimed professional status. The attributes of a profession include a unique body of knowledge, professional autonomy and self-governance, specialized education, research activities and contributions, and certification or other special recognition of its members. The word "professional" describes both a person and that person's demeanor. Core professional attributes and values include, among possible others, accountability, advocacy, altruism, autonomy, compassion, competence (technical and cultural), empathy, fiduciary status, loyalty, patience, social responsibility, staying focused under stress, team play, and truthfulness.

KEY WORDS AND PHRASES

- Advance directives
- Advocacy
- Affirmative action
- Allied health professional
- Altruism
- Appropriate
- Autonomy
- Business ethics

- Certification
- Charismatic power
- Code of ethics
- Coercive power
- Compassion
- Competence
- Comportment
- Conduct

- Countertransference
- Cultural competence
- Domain
- Empathy
- Expert
- Expertise
- Fee-for-service
- Fiduciary
- Health Insurance Portability and Accountability Act (HIPAA)
- Iatrogenic
- Industrial Revolution
- Informed consent
- Institutional ethics committee
- Introspection
- Jurisdiction
- Licensure
- Loyalty
- Managed care organization
- Nonmaleficence
- Nosocomial
- Novice
- Omission
- Organizational power
- Patient autonomy
- Patience
- Power
- Preauthorization
- Privilege
- *Pro bono publico* service
- Profession
- Professional
- Professional autonomy
- Professional ethics
- Professionalism
- Prognosis
- Prospective payment
- Protected health information
- Research
- Scope of practice
- Scope of personal competence
- Sharp debridement
- Significant other
- Social responsibility
- Standard of practice
- Stress
- Team play
- Technical competence
- Therapeutic privilege
- Transference
- Truthfulness
- Turf wars
- Variable incentive bonus

OBJECTIVES

1. Recognize and describe the three "classic" professions.
2. Evaluate the attributes that make someone a professional.
3. Define and distinguish patient and professional autonomy.
4. Analyze the named core professional values, and suggest other core professional values applicable to health care professionals.
5. Synthesize the recognized attributes and values of a professional into your health professional practice.

What Is a Profession?

Webster's dictionary defines a profession as "a whole body of persons engaged in a calling, vocation or employment." Put more clearly and precisely, a profession includes all members of a discipline that carry out the specialized work and service defined by that discipline and by society.

Historically, in Western societies, only three "classic" professions were recognized—attorneys at law, the clergy, and medical doctors. These three classes of workers were the first to be literate and the first to undergo university-level education. The exclusive "club" that they formed was elitist, racist, and sexist. Its members were almost exclusively wealthy white males. The monopoly that they held on higher education and professional status was backed by the power of the state at the macro level and by the guilds or colleges that they formed at the micro level. The Irish author George Bernard Shaw (1856–1950) called professions "conspiracies against the laity (masses)."

Power is defined as the ability to compel others to do your will, even against their own desires and interests. Types of power include organizational (hierarchal), coercive, charismatic, and power based on expertise. Classic professionals held (and may still hold to some degree) a great degree of power over others in society, based on their fundamental knowledge base and the vital roles that they play in society.

Over time, at least five attributes of a profession were developed. A profession may be characterized by the following:

- A defined and unique body of accrued knowledge and expertise, such that no one else is competent to carry out the professional roles and duties of its members.

- Autonomy, or self-governance, including the establishment of standards of practice for members and a code of ethics defining the official conduct of members.

- Formal education—especially including professional (entry-level) and post-professional higher education, training, and development—of its members.

- Research and other investigative and introspective activities designed to validate, refine, and improve its professional activities and services.

- Formal recognition of advanced member competency by certification or other processes.

Societies became less agrarian in the late 18th and 19th centuries as they became more urban and began to focus more and more on technology and occupational specialization. This Industrial Revolution led to many occupational groups claiming status as professionals. Although today the definition and parameters of a profession are less clear, it seems that many,

A profession includes all members of a discipline that carry out the specialized work and service defined by that discipline and by society.

many more occupations are professions than just law, medicine, and the clergy. All of the attributes of a profession may still be present, except that the first one—a unique body of accrued knowledge and expertise—has to be modified so that in an era of interdependence among complementary professions there are overlapping competence and expertise among professionals of different disciplines.

The defined knowledge base of a classic profession is what developed modernly into an exclusive "scope of practice." Modernly, this jurisdiction or practice domain established by a profession is often vigorously defended against intrusion in the courts and before legislatures and regulatory bodies when professionals from other disciplines seek to overlap that jurisdiction with their practices. This is especially true for select health professions.

What Is Professionalism?

There are two definitions for "professional." One definition describes a person who is a professional; one can also label the comportment (official behavior) of that person as professional or nonprofessional. A professional acts in a professional manner at all times while on the job.

According to Wikipedia, there is no definition for a modern professional; however, the modern professional possesses the following attributes. He or she

A professional acts in a professional manner at all times while on the job.

takes work seriously and carries it out expertly. The professional dresses appropriately for all business occasions and stays abreast of the latest developments in the field. She or he is client focused and cognizant of social responsibilities.

Consider the following exemplar. The Oregon Bar Association has a unique website entitled "Statement of Professionalism," devoted exclusively to expected behaviors of its member–attorneys. Its introduction reads as follows:

> As members of the Oregon State Bar, we belong to a profession devoted to serving both the interests of our clients and the public good. In our roles as officers of the court, as counselors, and as advocates, we aspire to a professional standard of conduct. With adherence to a professional standard of conduct, we earn a reputation for honor, respect, and trustworthiness among our clients, in the legal community, and with the public.

The Oregon Bar Association's professionalism website for attorneys also offers a description, if not a definition, of professionalism. It reads as follows:

> Professionalism includes integrity, honesty, and willing compliance with the highest ethical standards. Professionalism goes beyond observing the legal profession's ethical rules: professionalism sensitively and fairly serves the best interests of clients and the public. Professionalism fosters respect and trust among lawyers, and between lawyers and the public, promotes the efficient resolution of disputes, simplifies transactions, and makes the practice of law more enjoyable and satisfying.

Chapter Exercise 1

Access the Oregon Bar Association attorney–member professionalism webpage at www.osbar.org/rulesregs/professionalism. Read and analyze for clarity the 16 general professionalism guidelines for attorney conduct. How many of these standards can be applied directly to health care professionals?

What Makes a Health Care Professional Unique?

A health care professional is unique because of the nature of the work he or she performs and the status of the clients. In many cases, clinical health care delivery is emergent. Patients present themselves for care in life-and-death scenarios, and they and their families and significant others are often fearful or sad over possible outcomes of intervention.

Health care professionals care for patients 24 hours per day, 7 days per week, 365 days per year. Their clientele spans the lifespan continuum, from conception to old age. Most health care professionals deliver clinical services to patients and must stay abreast of ever-evolving information management systems, medications, procedures, and technology.

There are seven principal venues in which health care is practiced. Of the more than 0.5 million sites from which health care is delivered, three quarters are offices—outpatient facilities—managed by physicians or other primary health care providers. Hospitals—inpatient facilities—account for only 2% of the total number of health care facilities, but employ nearly half (40%) of all health care workers.

The other five venues for delivery of health care services include home health agencies; assisted living, skilled nursing, and long-term care facilities;

outpatient monitoring facilities, such as dialysis centers; laboratories; and diagnostic imaging centers.

According to the U.S. Department of Labor's Bureau of Labor Statistics, health care is the largest source of employment in the United States. In 2004, there were 13.5 million health care jobs—13.1 million jobs for wage-earning and salaried workers and about 411,000 self-employed positions. Eight of 20 occupations projected to grow the fastest over the next several years are in health care. More new wage and salary jobs—about 19%, or 3.6 million— created between 2004 and 2014 will be in health care than in any other occupational field.

Health care professionals tend to be older than workers in most other fields and remain in place because of the high levels of formal and informal education and training associated with their work. Shortages of qualified health care primary and support professionals will exacerbate as more

> Health care professionals are unique because of the nature of the work they perform and because of the status of their clients.

patients require care, large numbers of retirements ensue, and tighter immigration laws stem the entry of foreign-educated health care workers. This last trend will be blunted in part by increased outsourcing of selected health care work, particularly reading computerized diagnostic imaging studies, to professionals in foreign countries.

Core Professional Attributes and Values of a Health Professional

The core attributes and values of a health care professional are those that constitute the essence of everyday functioning of that professional. Everyone in health care delivery is a professional—support professionals, including assistants and aides; primary and consulting clinical professionals, such as occupational, physical, and speech therapists, primary care physicians and physician–specialists; clerical and administrative professionals; maintenance professionals; and a myriad of others.

Please avoid using the term "paraprofessional." In Greek, "para" means near, alongside, or beside. Support professionals in health care service delivery are professionals in their own right and deserve professional status and labeling. Please refer to them as support professionals.

Many health professional organizations and associations representing members of health care disciplines have developed lists of core values for members. For example, the American Physical Therapy Association came up with a list of seven core values for member physical therapists in 2000. They include accountability, altruism, compassion, excellence, integrity, professional duty, and social responsibility.

The following is my list of 14 core professional attributes and values for clinical health care professionals, developed over 36 years as a health care clinical professional, educator, and health law attorney.

Chapter Exercise 2

After perusing the list and descriptions of core professional attributes and values listed here, come up with personal additions to the list. Jot down descriptions and log personal exemplars about each in a journal to keep and add to as you enter and progress in practice.

Accountability

Conduct a Google search of the word accountability, and you will find categories of accountability like corporate, governmental, school, and social accountability. It seems that in every professional and social endeavor one is expected to be accountable for her or his conduct. That is true, especially for health care professionals.

Webster's dictionary defines accountability very briefly as being "responsible." Wikipedia offers a slightly broader description of accountability. It describes accountability as both an ethical and sociological concept. The sociological concept of accountable reportedly was first articulated in 1956 by Austin and expanded by Scott and Lyman in 1968.

Accountability is responsibility to oneself and others for one's conduct. Conduct includes affirmative actions undertaken by a professional or other individual, as well as omissions, actions consciously not undertaken. Accountability has ethical, legal, and sociological dimensions.

Under law, every person is accountable for his or her public conduct. At a minimum, everyone must act reasonably in public so as not to unreasonably harm any person or property. That basic legal "standard of care" is expanded for licensed professionals, especially health care professionals. Health care professionals, like airline pilots, architects, and attorneys at law, have the highest degree of legal accountability because they hold patients' lives in their hands. Their official conduct literally determines whether patients will live or die.

> Accountability is responsibility to oneself, others, and society for one's conduct.

Because of that fact, health care professionals at all levels of patient interaction must strive for practice excellence.

Advocacy

According to Answers.com's Free Dictionary, advocacy is the act of pleading or arguing in favor of something or someone. It entails active and vigorous support for a particular cause. We always think of a trial attorney as the archetypal advocate for legal clients in trouble. Wikipedia's definition of advocacy also includes collective organized activism in favor of political or social issues of interest.

An advocate then is a champion for a cause. Health care professionals are advocates for their patients and clients. On an everyday basis, health care professionals must advance their patients' interests to others—fellow health professionals who co-treat patients, administrators who make decisions about retention or discharge of patients, third-party (bill) payers (TPPs), patients' employers, and family members and significant others, whose personal interests may be in conflict with patients' best interests.

Chapter Exercise 3

Make a list of 10 persons or entities with whom health care professionals might need to be an advocate on a patient's behalf. Prioritize them on the basis of difficulty in winning over to your side of an issue (1 = most difficult to convince; 10 = least difficult to convince).

Consider the following hypothetical case example:

> A is an inpatient in ABC Hospital. A has metastatic breast cancer that has spread to her bones. A is terminal. She is expected to live only 3 to 6 more months. B, A's attending physician and rehabilitation team leader, has imposed *therapeutic privilege*, a gag order, disallowing other health professional team members from discussing A's prognosis with her. B believes that to discuss her condition with her will seriously jeopardize her current health and well-being. C is a licensed practical nurse caring for A. One day during bedside care, A asks C why her arm is hurting her so much when she walks with a walker. How should C respond?

> C is bound for the time being by B's invocation of therapeutic privilege, which is clearly written in the physician's orders in A's medical record. If C disagrees strongly with B's order, C should

1. Speak with B about it.
2. Discuss the issue at the next regularly scheduled or an *ad hoc* team meeting.
3. Call for assistance from the institutional ethics committee, a multidisciplinary committee within the facility that assists physicians and other health care professionals with ethical and moral problems, issues, and dilemmas.
4. Ask to withdraw from A's treatment team.

C is not free to discuss A's prognosis with A at this time; however, C should not lie to A and say that nothing is wrong. C simply must defer discussing the issue with A at the present time.

Another important area of advocacy for health care professionals involves advocating on patients' behalf for payment of charges for services by third-party payers (TPPs), or insurers. Managed care has caused TPPs to question and deny bills for health services more often than under the former fee-for-service payment system. Under managed care, there is prospective (lump sum) payment for most health care services provided to patients, making it difficult to obtain additional monies for additional services. Also, under managed care, many services and procedures require preauthorization from TPPs before services can be rendered. Additional reasons for denial of payment by TPPs include "lack of medical necessity" and "experimental treatment."

When bills for health services have been denied by TPPs, health care providers must seek reconsideration through carefully drafted appeals. Appeals often must be processed through several levels, and thus, they are time consuming and require precision. Many articles and websites offer free help for drafting and processing claims denial appeals, and thus, there is no excuse for not advocating for payment for services on patients' behalf after denial. Otherwise, patients themselves will be billed for many of these services.

> An advocate is a champion for a cause. Health care professionals are advocates for their patients and clients.

Altruism

According to Dic.die.net, altruism means displaying unselfish concern for the welfare of others. In the case of health care professionals at all levels of service, altruism describes the value of seeking to do the best possible for patients and clients.

Don Quixote was the personification of altruism. The 15th-century Spanish knight-errant saw beauty and good in everything and everyone that he encountered. He also strove to right wrongs wherever he saw them. The term "quixotic" came to mean idealistic and impractical.

Health care professionals, like teachers and a select few others, are instinctively quixotic, or at least half quixotic. (Although they may be idealistic, they cannot afford to be impractical, especially under managed care.) Health care professionals routinely put their own health and well-being on the line for the patients they care for. Patients come first. Under an altruistic health care delivery model, they always have and always will.

> The altruist displays unselfish concern for the welfare of others. The health professional altruist seeks always to do the best possible for patients and clients under care.

Health care is not just another business. When patients' lives hang daily in the balance, it cannot be treated as such.

Managed care, with its primary focus on cost-containment, makes it more difficult to practice altruism. It is necessarily more difficult (but not impossible) to do the best for patients when the system demands cost-minimization.

The epitome of altruism is *pro bono publico* service. *Pro bono* service entails providing needed health services at low or no cost to socioeconomically disadvantaged patients and clients. Many, but not all, health care disciplines address *pro bono* patient care services in their ethics codes and/or other core documents. More can and must be done to address the health care needs of patients lacking the ability to pay for services.

Attorneys at law perhaps have the most extensive record of *pro bono* service of any profession. In many states, including Texas, licensed attorneys must account annually in writing for their *pro bono* activities upon renewal of their licenses.

Chapter Exercise 4

Investigate any state bar association's webpage, and examine it for *pro bono* service activities for member attorneys at law. Which attorney expectations can be directly adapted for immediate use by health care professional disciplines?

Autonomy

The Greek word autonomy means auto- or self-law, the right to govern oneself. Modernly, autonomy refers to self-governance and self-determination.

The law and health professional ethics codes have long given adult patients who possess full mental capacity the right of autonomy over their bodies and over what medical treatments can be done to and for them. The law and ethics of informed consent are centered on respect for patient autonomy over health care decision making.

For patients lacking legal (minors) or mental capacity, the law and health professional ethics codes assign autonomy over treatment decision making to surrogate decision makers, such as parents, guardians, or agents acting under durable health care powers of attorney. Patients are free to appoint such guardians or agents pursuant to advance directives, which, like living wills, delineate patients' wishes regarding health care interventions in the event of their incapacitation.

Patients are not the only persons within the health care system to have autonomy. Health care providers, organizations, and systems also possess autonomy. Such autonomy is called professional autonomy.

Professional autonomy means that health care professionals are free to practice within wide parameters of acceptable practice, according to their beliefs, education, and experiences. They are free in a capitalistic society such as the United States to practice individually or in groups (depending on their disciplines) or to be employed in hospitals or by health systems. Health care professionals are free to charge for services anywhere along a broad continuum of reasonable fees for services without violating the law or ethics provisions.

> Professional autonomy gives health care providers the right to exercise independent professional judgment to best serve their patients' needs.

Compassion and Empathy

Compassion is a core attribute of health care professionals. Compassion entails a deep awareness of other peoples' suffering, coupled with a strong desire to help relieve it. It includes caring concern and empathy for patients and their well-being.

Empathy means putting oneself in another's place. You never really understand a person's problems until you walk a mile in his or her shoes. Empathy differs from sympathy in that being sympathetic does not require the sympathizer to buy into a person's pain, just to be sad about it. Sympathy merely means feeling sorry for someone. It is a passive versus active state of mind.

Medical technology and other advances, sophisticated information management systems, and new models for health care delivery integration like managed care do not change the fact that it is simple human compassion and empathy, manifested through a genuinely warm human touch, that makes health care uniquely special.

If anyone that I have ever known personifies compassion toward patients, it is Mr. Tomas Moreno. I had the privilege to work with Tomas at Health-South-Crestway in San Antonio, Texas during 2004 and 2005. I was the newly appointed physical therapist in charge, and Tomas was the rehabilitation aide for the clinic. Tomas had worked in his position at HealthSouth-Crestway for nearly a decade when I arrived. He bore a huge administrative and clinical support burden—always with a smile. As the sole support professional on site, Tomas worked with in support of all of the occupational, physical, and speech therapists—employees and contractors—in the clinic. He was also the clinic's Spanish translator for Mexican and Mexican-American patients. His patients loved him, and so did the staff and all official visitors to the clinic. He had a motto that I tried to adopt as my own: "Treat patients like gold and spoil them rotten." Patients seemed to get better quicker and with less pain because of Tomas' caring, empathetic attitude and great sense of humor. No one did it better than Tomas. He retired shortly after I left the clinic in June 2005.

> Compassion and empathy are attributes that give health care professionals tools to more effectively serve their patients' needs.

Competence

Competence refers to one's capability to carry out the critical and ancillary roles of one's job. For health care professionals, knowledge of the parameters of the job is crucial for optimal patient welfare. Patients' lives literally hang in the balance every day. When health care professionals are not working at peak competency, iatrogenic (provider caused) injuries and nosocomial (health care facility acquired) infections ensue.

> There are three learning domains: cognitive (acquisition of knowledge), psychomotor (hands-on skills), and affective (one's comportment or behavior). For health care professionals at all levels, all three domains are critically important.

Health care professionals gain new competence and insight continuously. They learn enough in their professional (entry-level) formal education programs to qualify for licensing or certification examinations, or registry, as applicable. They may undertake clinical affiliations or internships that help to develop their psychomotor skills as well as their cognitive and affective skill sets.

After they graduate from formal education programs, health care professionals are novices—new to their fields and without a great deal of experience. Through months and years of experience and additional formal and informal education, training, and development, they mature into expert clinicians.

These health professional experts think schematically, as in a matrix, short cutting what was formerly for them a lengthy decision making process, quickly coming up with accurate diagnoses and optimal interventions for their patients.

There are two domains of competence. Technical competence is the ability to execute the requisites of one's job efficiently and effectively. Health care professionals must be able and willing to admit when certain tasks are beyond their scope of personal competence or their legal scope of practice. Consider the following exemplar:

> Q is a staff physical therapist at XYZ Medical Center. Q is treating R, a patient with a diabetic foot ulcer, at bedside. S, a contract podiatrist who has only limited time to see a high volume of patients at the facility, directs Q to carry out light, sharp debridement of R's diabetic foot ulcer. Q is a new graduate and has no experience doing sharp debridement. How should Q proceed?

> Q should immediately inform S that sharp debridement is beyond Q's scope of personal competence and should not attempt to carry out S's directive. The ethical concept of nonmaleficence disallows causing intentional harm to patients, which following S's order would result in. Q should find a more experienced co-staff physical therapist to carry out the procedure ordered by S. (Note that the procedure is within the legal scope of practice for physical therapists under most or all state practice acts.)

In addition to technical competence, health care professionals have a duty in a multicultural society such as the United States to be culturally competent as well. Cultural competence entails recognizing and accommodating disparate beliefs, customs, mores, and practices of members of a multicultural society having diverse backgrounds.

Health care law expressly takes patients' diverse backgrounds and languages into account in many instances. For example, the law of patient informed consent requires health care providers to communicate the parameters of informed disclosure to patients in languages that they understand. Similarly, the privacy provisions of the Health Insurance Portability and Accountability Act (HIPAA) require that patients be informed of their protected health information privacy rights in their operative languages before physical examination and the commencement of care. These topics are discussed further in Chapter 4.

> *Technical competence* is the ability to execute the requisites of one's job efficiently and effectively. *Cultural competence* is the recognition and accommodation of disparate beliefs and practices of members of a multicultural society having diverse backgrounds.

Fiduciary Status

The concept of a fiduciary is an ancient Roman law concept. A fiduciary is a person who is charged by law to put the interests of another person above his or her own interests, within the confines of his or her official relationship. In such a relationship, the fiduciary is a trustee, and the person whose interests predominate is called a beneficiary. All health care professionals are fiduciaries to their patients.

> A fiduciary is a person charged by law to put the interests of another person above his or her own interests. Health care professionals are fiduciaries to their patients.

In everyday clinical practice, health professionals face multiple conflicting interests, particularly personal and practice concerns such as financial self-interest. Consider the following hypothetical example and answer the question posed.

X is a physician who is employed by CDE Managed Care Organization. X carries out over 5,000 patient visits per year in an outpatient setting. A portion of X's compensation package includes a variable incentive bonus. The condition for payment of this bonus is that X must reduce last year's average total cost of care per patient from $75 to $65. If this is accomplished, CDE and X then split the $50,000 savings realized 50-50. What is the potential ethical problem with this scheme?

Loyalty

Loyalty is a core value that is closely akin to being a fiduciary. In the case of the fiduciary–beneficiary relationship, the health professional and patient are the participants. In the hypothetical example posed previously, the variable incentive bonus may cause X to compromise the patients' care by shaving costs too deeply. X may place her or his own financial interests above the health care interests of patients under care. When one is a fiduciary, this outcome is prohibited by law and ethics.

X should reflect on the situation and make the following disclosure to patients:

> Part of my compensation includes variable incentive pay for reducing costs paid by my employer, CDE. In the process of attempting to reduce costs, I promise not to compromise optimal quality health care delivery to you or to any other patient.

Health care professionals owe multiple loyalties to multiple persons and entities. Although health care professionals owe their pre-eminent duty to patients under care, they also owe duties of loyalty to their employers. Part of the duty owed to employers includes the duty not to appropriate (steal) patients for their own private practices once they leave employment. This legal duty exists even in the absence of any express contractual promise not to appropriate patients.

> Loyalty means fidelity or faithful adherence to obligations to others. The highest duty owed by health care professionals is to patients under their immediate care.

Health care professionals also owe duties of loyalty, or fidelity, to partners in group practices, to their professional associations and societies, and to their families and significant others. None of these duties, however, supersedes the highest duty owed to patients under care.

Patience and Staying Focused Under Stress

It is often said that "patience is a virtue." This proverb originated in *Piers Plowman* by William Langland in 1377. The virtue of patience entails remaining calm, restrained, and self-controlled in the face of delay or other impediments to accomplishment of one's mission. Sometimes it seems that health care professionals, beset by multiple simultaneous crises, must possess the patience of Job.

> Patience entails remaining calm, restrained, and self-controlled (calm, cool, and collected) in the face of delay or other impediments to accomplishment of one's mission.

Think about times when you have been a passenger on an airplane. Have you ever experienced a delay in taking off or landing at an airport? Of course you have. Who are the only people who do not become agitated by such delays? The flight crew. An impatient pilot is a danger to self and others. So is an impatient health care professional a danger to patients under care.

Social Responsibility

The modern usage for the term *social responsibility* in business originated in the 1980s. For the first time in U.S. history, the purposes of business were said to include not only the generation of net revenue, but also a strong commitment to society and its people. Businesses in a sociocapitalist society such as the United States are simply not free to pursue unbridled *laissez faire* profits but must balance revenue generation with a special formal duty owed to society and its inhabitants—citizens and noncitizens.

Social responsibility entails concern for society and its people and positive actions in support of that concern, especially for the disadvantaged. Health care professionals, like other licensed professionals, have a strong duty of social responsibility.

According to a recent Parade survey, nearly all (89%) middle-class Americans believe that businesses in the United States have a fundamental duty of social responsibility toward their communities and employees. Eighty-one percent of the same survey respondents also believe that businesses put their own interests, especially profits, ahead of their employees and the communities that support them.

Licensed health care professionals are privileged and sanctioned by law to invade a patient's intimate physical and mental spaces as part of their official duties. That privilege carries with it significant responsibility. There is strong sentiment, as reflected in the writings of economists Kleiner and Krueger, that professional licensing is overdone. They argue that the extra costs borne by patients and clients associated with paying for their providers' licensure may not be worth the expenditure. They also proffer that quality of service delivery is not substantially improved because providers are licensed.

Health care professionals interact with patients and clients at several physical distances, including the following:

1. Business or social distance for ordinary interpersonal exchanges, such as greeting one another or, in the case of health care professionals and patients, taking a patient history.

2. Personal distance, as when carrying out a patient examination.

3. Intimate distance, as when examining a patient in or on her or his private spaces.

As was stated in Chapter 1, health care professionals must, in all cases, use their best clinical judgment and skills to effect optimal therapeutic results for their patients. They are not free to violate patient confidentiality, absent some legal exception or excuse, such as a court order to reveal the information. Similarly, health care professionals must not take advantage of patients financially or sexually within their official provider–patient relationships.

The psychological concept of transference refers to situations in which patients transfer childlike emotions, including romantic affection, to persons in authority, such as treating health care professionals. Health care professionals are not permitted to respond in kind to displays of patient affection. Such countertransference is prohibited by professional codes of ethics and state statutes, administrative regulations, and case law governing health care practice.

In addition to providing *pro bono* services to patients in need, companies—including health care organizations—are showing social responsibility by encouraging their employees to volunteer their time and services in the community. According to Knight, 35% of nonprofit executives believe that volunteerism is key to improving the corporate bottom line. Because social responsibility enhances business goodwill as well as serves a noble purpose, it allows companies and individuals to "do well while doing good."

> Social responsibility entails concern for society and its people and positive actions in support of that concern, especially for the disadvantaged.

Team Play

The importance of the health care interdisciplinary team has already been discussed in detail in Chapter 1. The core value of team play means that health care professionals at all levels must subordinate personal interests, attention, and gain in favor of their teams' efforts in support of patients and their welfare.

For several decades, the term allied health professional has been in vogue to describe most health care providers who work together with physicians and nurses for patients' benefit. Included as allied health professionals are occupational, physical, and speech therapists; orthotists and prosthetists; laboratory technologists; and many others. Because the term allied health took on the secondary connotation of "ancillary" versus essential, some health care disciplines began to object to being labeled allied health professions.

> Team play means that health professionals at all levels subordinate personal interests, attention, and gain in favor of their teams' efforts in support of patients and their welfare. This is the essence of patient-focused care.

The better approach is to consider all health care professionals to be allied health care professionals, that is, allied in teams in support of patients they care for. Under this definition, everyone from a surgeon to a nurse to a physical therapist to an x-ray technician to a nurses' aide is an allied health professional. The purpose of patient-focused care is to divert the focus from individual health care providers and their interests exclusively toward patients and their welfare. The whole is only as good as the sum of its parts.

Truthfulness

The final core value in the alphabetized list of 14 is truthfulness. If ever the adage "last but not least" was apropos, this is the time. Optimal health care delivery to patients requires truthfulness on the part of its team members virtually all of the time. Patients put their lives in the hands of their treating health care providers largely because they know that they can trust them to be truthful—particularly about patients' diagnoses, prognoses, and privacy interests.

> Truthfulness is more than being honest and straightforward with others. It also includes being authentic and genuine—the "real deal."

Truthfulness includes more than just honesty and veracity in dealing with others. The trait of truthfulness also entails authenticity and genuineness. Truthfulness on the part of one person engenders confidence in others about their relationships with that person.

The legal health care professional–patient privilege safeguards almost anything said by patients to their physicians, psychotherapists, and other primary health care providers. This legal privilege, in states where it applies, prevents health care professionals from being compelled to reveal in legal proceedings most confidential information revealed to them by patients during the care relationship.

Another rare exception to truthfulness is therapeutic privilege. Therapeutic privilege is a legal concept under which a physician head of a health care team may write an order imposing a gag order on team members, disallowing them from revealing diagnostic or prognostic information to select patients. This is done because the physician believes that such patients cannot psychologically handle information about their diagnoses and/or prognoses.

> Fourteen core professional attributes and values for clinical health care professionals are as follows:
>
> 1. Accountability
> 2. Advocacy
> 3. Altruism
> 4. Autonomy
> 5. Compassion
> 6. Competence
> 7. Empathy
> 8. Fiduciary status
> 9. Loyalty
> 10. Patience
> 11. Social responsibility
> 12. Staying focused under stress
> 13. Team play
> 14. Truthfulness

In situations in which a team member disagrees with such an order, the team member may exercise a range of options, from discussing it with the physician to calling a meeting of the treating team to invoking the aid of the institutional ethics committee. Because therapeutic privilege derogates from respect for patient autonomy, it is rarely invoked by physicians and even more rarely allowed to stand by courts of law.

QUESTIONS AND CASES FOR STUDY

1. What is the exclusive defined body of knowledge and expertise for clergy, lawyers, and doctors that qualifies them for "classic professional" status? Modernly, which other professionals, if any, encroach on (overlap) their formerly exclusive occupational jurisdictions? Has such encroachment harmed or improved the quality of services delivered by these classic professionals?

2. What type(s) of power do health care professionals exercise over patients and clients and their significant others—organizational (hierarchal), coercive, charismatic, or power based on expertise? What role does patient autonomy (supremacy) over treatment decision making have, if any, in altering the power dynamics of the health professional–patient relationship?

3. What can health care professionals do—individually and collectively—to help meet the formidable *pro bono* health care services needs of socioeconomically disadvantaged patients and clients in the United States?

4. Health professional education programs evaluate students' levels of empathy during simulations and clinical instruction. Can you teach someone to be empathetic? Is this an affective skill that can be learned and refined?

5. A Vietnamese-speaking patient arrives for care at your private practice clinic. No one on staff speaks Vietnamese. How can you obtain informed consent and communicate with the patient? (Hint: see references 7, 21, and 22.)

REFERENCES, READINGS, AND RESOURCES

1. Austin JL. 1956–7. A plea for excuses. Proceedings of the Aristotelian Society. Reprinted in JO Urmson & GJ Warnock, eds., 3rd ed. J.L. Austin: Philosophical Papers, Oxford: Clarendon Press, 1979, 175–204.

2. *Black's Law Dictionary*, 5th ed. St. Paul: West Publishing Group, 1979.

3. Cavasar J. Origin of 'Patience is a Virtue.' www.originofphrases.org.uk (May 12, 2000).

4. Cervantes Saavedra M. *El Ingenioso Hidalgo Don Quijote de la Mancha.* de la Cuesta: Madrid, Spain, 1605, 1615.

5. Early C, Mosakowski E. Cultural intelligence. *Harvard Business Review.* Oct. 2004, 139–146.

6. Fandray D. Values matter: Decision making is more than choosing between right and wrong. *Continental Magazine.* Sept. 2005, 82–84.

7. Kaplan M. Wie sagt man . . . ? Sites that'll translate anything. *USA Weekend.* Oct. 8–10, 2004, 16.

8. Kleiner MM. *Licensing Occupations: Ensuring Quality or Restricting Competition.* Kalamazoo, MI: Upjohn Institute, 2006.

9. Knight D. Giving back. *Indianapolis Star.* Apr. 30, 2006, D1, D8.

10. Krueger AB. Do you need a license to earn a living? You might be surprised about the answer. *New York Times.* Mar. 2, 2006, C3.

11. Langland W. *Piers Plowman.* Dublin: Trinity College (ms212), 1377.

12. Leonhardt D, Bajaj V. U.S. economy is still growing at rapid pace. *New York Times.* April 28, 2006, A1, C4.

13. Scott MB, Lyman SM. Accounts. *American Sociological Review.* 1968;33:46–62.

14. Scott RW. *Legal Aspects of Documenting Patient Care for Rehabilitation Professionals,* 3rd ed. Sudbury, MA: Jones and Bartlett, 2006.

15. Scott RW. *Professional Ethics: A Guide for Rehabilitation Professionals.* St. Louis: Mosby, 1997.

16. *Webster's Ninth New Collegiate Dictionary.* Springfield, MA: Merriam-Webster, 1985.

17. *Wikipedia: The Free Encyclopedia.* En.wikipedia.org. Accessed April 16, 2006.

18. www.Answers.com (Free Dictionary)

19. www.appliedautonomy.com (Institute for Applied Autonomy. See free video—Bridging the Gap)

20. www.apta.org (American Physical Therapy Association)

21. www.freetranslation.com (medical translation assistance)

22. www.languageline.com (AT&T's confidential medical translation service)

23. www.dic.die.net

24. www.healthsymphony.com (appealing medical claims denials)

25. www.osbar.org/rulesregs/professionalism.htm (Oregon Bar Association)

26. www.texasbar.com (Texas Bar Association)

Chapter 3

Morals, Ethics, and the Law: Your Special Duties Owed to Patients and to the Health Care System

ABSTRACT

Health care providers are often torn between and among conflicting senses of duty—moral duty, ethical duty, and legal duty. They must always comply with each of the aforementioned duties in their practices. Modernly, legal and professional ethical obligations have become blurred or blended, in part because people have become increasingly litigious. Health care professionals have the responsibility to be cognizant of key laws and regulations governing their practices. These areas of law include, among possible others, health care malpractice, informed consent, legal aspects of patient care documentation, privacy, and relevant business, contractual, criminal, and employment law concepts. All health care professionals need to assimilate into practice a systematic method for identifying and resolving ethical problems, issues, and dilemmas that inevitably arise. The systems model is one such easy-to-apply method.

KEY WORDS AND PHRASES

- Active euthanasia
- Americans with Disabilities Act
- Breach of contract
- Business law
- Case law
- Collateral source rule
- Comparative fault
- Constitutional law

- Criminal law
- Deposition
- Diplomatic immunity
- Equity
- Ethical duty
- Expert witness
- Ethical decision making framework
- Health Care Insurance Portability and Accountability Act
- Health care malpractice
- Informed consent
- Intentional misconduct
- Interrogatory
- Joint and several liability
- Jurisdiction
- Legal duty
- Moral duty
- National Practitioner Data Bank
- Occupational Safety and Health Act

- Ordinary negligence
- Pain and suffering
- Patient abandonment
- Patient care documentation
- Precedent
- Problem, issue, dilemma
- Professional corporation
- Professional negligence
- Regulatory law
- *Res ipsa loquitur*
- *Stare decisis*
- Standard of care
- State practice act
- Statute of limitations
- Statute of repose
- Strict product liability
- Supremacy
- Systems model
- Tort reform
- Vicarious liability

OBJECTIVES

1. Define and distinguish moral, ethical, and legal duties in clinical health care practice.
2. Analyze the modern blending or mixing of health law and professional ethics.
3. Synthesize the law and ethics of patient informed consent universally into clinical practice at all levels.
4. Understand the law of health care malpractice and practice effective risk management to minimize malpractice exposure in practice.
5. Practice effective patient care documentation that meets all organizational and legal requirements.
6. Develop, implement, and refine, as needed, a lifelong personal approach to professional ethical decision making.

Moral, Ethical, and Legal Duties Defined and Distinguished

Morals are personal beliefs, mores, practices, and standards that influence or govern individuals' lives. Morals are often, but not exclusively, grounded in one's religious convictions. At the base level of conduct, a person acts according to moral beliefs.

Ethics involve organized rules of conduct governing a person's official conduct. The classic professions of the law, medicine, and the clergy have had in place codes of ethics for millennia. Health professional codes of ethics are among the most comprehensive and well-developed and refined codes of ethical conduct.

State practice acts, which are part of regulatory laws governing health care practice, are based in large part on codes of ethics. The provisions they contain often closely mirror professional association codes of ethics. Regulatory law is also known as administrative law. Professionals, including health care providers, have the most interface with regulatory agencies and personnel. Examples of federal regulatory agencies include the Equal Employment Opportunity Commission (EEOC), the Internal Revenue Service (IRS), and the Occupational Safety and Health Administration (OSHA). State-level administrative agencies include, among others, health professional licensing boards and state insurance commissions.

Chapter Exercise 1

Access your discipline's professional association website, and examine its code of ethics. Select another complementary health care discipline, and examine its professional code of ethics. Compare the two codes of ethics. How are they similar? How are they different, if at all?

Legal obligations bind nearly everyone in society to its provisions and mandates. Without a strong legal system in place, there would be chaos in any society. Think of Iraq after the fall of Saddam Hussein. The anarchy and lack of civility between and among ethnic and religious factions in Iraq could not be reversed, even under martial law imposed by the United States, Great Britain, and other occupying coalition nations.

Virtually everyone is subject to obey the law. Only one class of persons is technically "above the law." Who are they? No, not the President,

> Without a strong legal system in place, there would be chaos in any society.

Vice-President, and members of Congress. Technically, international diplomats are the only persons immune from legal processes, under the complex concept of diplomatic immunity. Diplomatic immunity belongs, however, not to individual diplomats, but to the nation-states they represent. After being charged with a crime in a country where a diplomat (or her or his family) is stationed, the country of origin can waive diplomatic immunity and allow the criminal suspect to be prosecuted under local law. The primary rationale in favor of diplomatic immunity is that, without it, U.S. diplomats and their staff and families would be subject to harassment, malicious prosecution, and even imprisonment while stationed in unfriendly countries.

> Active euthanasia: intentional conduct (action or inaction [omission]) designed to end a person's suffering by ending that person's life—assisted suicide.

Acting according to one's morals may not conform to ethical or legal standards in all cases. For example, even if a health professional's personal beliefs permitted him or her to carry out active euthanasia (assisted suicide) on another person, health professional ethical and legal standards would not so permit. That is why morals, ethics, and law act, not only in concert, but also as checks and balances on one another.

> Morals, ethics, and law act, not only in concert, but also as checks and balances on one another.

Similarly, even when conduct is legal and permissible under applicable codes of ethics and practice standards, an individual health care professional should never compromise personal moral standards and engage in conduct prohibited by such moral standards. For example, even where elective abortion is legal, no health care provider can be compelled to take part in such a procedure if it is contrary to his or her moral beliefs.

Chapter Exercise 2

Develop a hypothetical case example describing a mixed moral, ethical, and legal problem, issue, or dilemma from health care clinical practice. How would you resolve the problem presented? If you are in a classroom setting, share your hypothetical case and resolution with your colleagues.

The Modern Blending of Health Law and Ethics

Although legal and health professional ethical obligations seemingly involve distinct duties incumbent on health care providers, they have in fact become enmeshed in modern times. What now constitutes a breach of legal duties by health care professionals almost always also constitutes a breach of professional ethics. This modern blending of health law and professional ethics is like a partial eclipse of the Sun, with near-total overlap of the two spheres of law and ethics.

Modern legal and ethical standards developed, in large part, from rulings by medieval law, ecclesiastical and equity courts within the British Commonwealth system. The sovereign's law courts, or "King's bench," strictly enforced written statutory laws, with little regard for morals or fairness. Courts of special jurisdiction enforced moral standards (ecclesiastical courts) and tried to provide fundamental fairness to participants (equity courts) within this complex legal system.

Historically, ecclesiastical courts reviewed church-related matters affecting members of the general public, including the fact and validity of marriage and questions of legitimacy. As Dan Brown correctly noted in *The Da Vinci Code*, ecclesiastical courts still exist today, although their jurisdiction is sharply limited, mainly to church hierarchy.

Equity courts in medieval times heard private civil disputes that could not be readily resolved in the law courts. Medieval equity courts were the first courts to hear *pro bono* cases brought on behalf of citizens too poor to pay for legal services.

Over time, ecclesiastical courts lost their power of general jurisdiction over the masses, and equity courts were melded into the legal system. This blending of law and ethics meant that, for the first time, judges were charged not only to enforce the law but also to seek to be fair to all litigants.

Part of the rationale for the modern blending of health law and professional ethics relates to the fact that people in modern societies are highly litigious. Tens of million lawsuits are filed annually in the United States alone.

Citizens (litigants) also are better educated, possess a well-developed sense of consumerism and entitlement, and are well-acclimated to the legal culture, in part through constant exposure in the media. The process of filing claims and complaints against licensed health care professionals to professional associations for alleged breaches is closely akin to that of filing a lawsuit or making a general claim to a regulatory agency. In summary, modern people in postmodern cultures are ready, willing, and able to assert and enforce their legal rights.

Sources of Legal and Ethical Duties

Legal obligations bind everyone in a society to obey "the rules." Even diplomats are not fully immune from legal processes if their host nations waive diplomatic immunity. Health care professional codes of ethics are promulgated through state licensing boards and professional associations. They address professional conduct and formally obligate health care professionals to comply with their provisions.

There are five sources of legal obligation. The highest order source of legal duty is the U.S. Constitution, particularly its Bill of Rights and subsequent amendments to the body of the Constitution. These amendments address personal rights and duties. One important constitutional right directly affecting health care professionals is the implied right of privacy, which was created by the U.S. Supreme Court in 1965 in the legal case *Griswold v. Connecticut*. That case ruled for the first time that a federal constitutional right of marital privacy existed, within which the government could not intrude. Over time, that right was extended to encompass individual autonomy in general and to elective abortion in 1973 in *Roe v. Wade*.

State constitutions may afford greater personal liberties and protections to state residents than does the federal Constitution; however, they are subordinate to the federal Constitution when the two documents' provisions are in conflict. This concept is called a "conflict of laws" issue.

Statutes, enacted by Congress and state legislatures, are subordinate to state and federal constitutions and their legal mandates. Here, we do not say that state statutes are necessarily subordinate to federal statutes, as the federal government (supposedly) has a very limited jurisdiction, or domain of power—exclusively over such areas as antitrust, bankruptcy, and military law issues. Most other areas, including regulation of professions and health care malpractice, are under near-exclusive state control.

Examples of federal statutes important to health care professionals include, among many others, the Americans with Disabilities Act (ADA), the Health Insurance Portability and Accountability Act (HIPAA), and the Occupational Safety and Health Act (OSHA).

Examples of state statutes important to health care professionals include statutes creating health professional practice acts, state insurance statutes, and business law statutes, such as those delineating the creation of professional corporations and those governing partnerships.

Case law decisions rendered by state and federal judges are subordinate in the hierarchy of legal authority to constitutional and statutory laws. Most health care malpractice law is judge-made case law. Case law remains relatively stable because of a concept called *stare decisis*, or let the decision stand. Judges are not free to overrule each other willy-nilly, but must conform to prior case decisions (called "precedent"), unless such rulings are over-turned by the highest court (usually called a supreme court) within a system.

Regulatory law, promulgated by administrative agencies, is the final source of primary legal authority. Regulatory or administrative law, created by governmental agencies at federal, state, and local levels, makes up the most pervasive source of legal duty. Health care providers have the greatest legal interface with regulatory agencies governing their practice. Examples of federal regulatory agencies include the EEOC, the IRS, and the OSHA. State agencies include education coordinating boards and health professions licensing boards. A zoning commission is an example of a local regulatory agency.

Chapter Exercise 3

Make a list of at least five regulatory agencies at federal, state, and local levels that directly or indirectly affect health care professionals. Describe what each agency does.

The fifth source of legal duty derives from secondary legal authorities, which although not laws in and of themselves, are influential to legal decision makers. Such things as accreditation body rules and regulations, health professional codes of ethics, and professional practice guidelines and protocols are examples of secondary or indirect legal authorities.

Select Health Professional Legal and Ethical Provisions and Applications

Health Care Malpractice Crisis

For the past few decades, the United States has experienced what has been labeled a health care malpractice crisis, characterized by large numbers of legal actions and larger civil malpractice verdicts in favor of patient–plaintiffs and against health care providers. This phenomenon has affected every health care professional that provides direct patient care services, including nurse practitioners, physical and occupational therapists, and physician assistants, among many others.

Direct health care providers face a high degree of malpractice exposure, not only because they treat patients when they are most at risk—sick or injured and often in pain—but also because of many other factors. External factors that increase providers' malpractice exposure include a greater sense of consumerism among the patient population, intensified federal and state regulation of health care delivery, and a metamorphosis in the health care milieu away from informal, personalized care in favor of increasingly competitive "business-like" delivery of health care.

Some health care disciplines have undergone substantive internal professional changes that may increase their members' health care malpractice liability risk exposure by making them more prominent in the public eye. Some of the internal factors that may create greater legal risks for providers within these disciplines specifically include the expanding scope and breadth of professional practice, the trends toward direct access practice or practice without physician referral in more and more jurisdictions, clinical specialty certification, and the publication of practice guidelines.

Obviously, not all health care malpractice claims and legal actions are frivolous. There are a substantial number of medical mistakes annually that result in serious bodily injury to or the death of patients. The Institute of Medicine, a Washington, D.C.-based nongovernmental organization focused on health, reported in 1999 that there are approximately 100,000 such medical "mistakes" involving hospitalized patients per year. In 2004, Health-Grades, a Colorado-based private entity that assesses the quality of health care delivery, doubled that number to 200,000. Although not all medical mistakes constitute health care malpractice, many do.

Health care malpractice plaintiffs do not prevail in their legal cases as often as they lose. On average, patient–plaintiffs prevailed in their lawsuits against health care providers in 2002 42% of the time. A 2001 study conducted by the U.S. Department of Justice found that in the 75 largest counties in the United States, patient–plaintiffs won health care malpractice cases only 27% of the time. Jury verdict dollar values, however, continue to rise. The median jury verdict in medical malpractice cases in 2002 was $1,018.86, according to Jury Verdict Research.

Health care professionals and clinical managers can do many things in practice to minimize the incidence of claims of health care malpractice and malpractice lawsuits. Of paramount importance is excellence in communications between health care providers and patients and among health care providers treating patients. In communicating with patients, providers must remember to explain what they are doing during clinical examinations. Providers also must explain examination and diagnostic test results to patients and explain them in simple lay person's language. Patients not only want information about their health status and care but are also entitled to it as a universal legal principle and fundamental human right. Under the legal concept of informed consent, health care providers must convey to patients sufficient information about their health status to allow patients to make informed choices about whether to accept or decline recommended interventions. Effective clinical documentation of primary provider–patient communication processes, especially regarding informed consent, is crucial to managing malpractice risk exposure.

In addition to effective communication with patients, health care providers must also communicate effectively and systematically with other health care professionals who are either concurrently treating a given patient or who will treat that patient in the future. The principal means of communicating information among health care providers is through patient care documentation. Accurate, timely, thorough, and concise documentation can be the deciding factor for whether a patient lives or dies. Effective documentation also has "professional" life-and-death consequences for health care providers charged with malpractice. In a malpractice trial, tried perhaps many years after care was rendered, what is written in the treatment record may constitute the only objective evidence of whether care given to a patient–plaintiff by a malpractice health professional–defendant met or breached minimally acceptable practice standards.

> Effective documentation in the treatment record may constitute the only objective evidence of whether care given to a patient by a health care professional met practice standards or was substandard.

Besides effective communication and documentation, other strategies can be used to help lessen the risk of malpractice actions. These include simple things such as treating patients with empathy and compassion, practicing only within one's personal scope of clinical competence and within the legal parameters of one's profession, consulting with other health care providers whenever necessary, and establishing within health care facilities effective quality and risk-management programs to monitor and evaluate patient care and to manage malpractice risk exposure.

Reflective of these considerations, legal issues concerning nonphysician health care specialties have received greater attention by legal and health care authors in the recent past. Professional associations, including, among others, the American Health Lawyers Association, the American Medical Association, the American Nurses Association, the American Occupational Therapy Association, and the American Physical Therapy Association, are sponsoring more professional seminars on selected legal topics such as risk management, expert testimony, and the legal standard of care.

Malpractice Defined

Legal writers and scholars have used two approaches to defining health care malpractice. Under the traditional approach, the definition of health care malpractice includes only conduct that constitutes professional negligence—the overwhelming basis for imposition of malpractice liability. Under a broader approach, however, every potential legal basis for imposition of health care malpractice liability—including professional negligence, breach of a therapeutic contractual promise made by a provider to a patient, patient or client injury from dangerously defective care-related equipment or other products (strict product liability), strict (absolute, non–fault-based) liability for abnormally dangerous care-related activities, and patient or client injury that results from intentional provider misconduct in the course of patient care—may be included in the definition of health care malpractice.

Most of these bases of malpractice liability—negligence, intentional conduct, and product and strict liability—are classified as "torts" (French for "wrongs"), a class of legal actions that encompasses most personal injuries except those caused by breach of contract. Torts are classified as private actions because they involve injuries personal to private parties, in contrast to crimes, which are public actions, or wrongs against society as a whole.

The broad definition of health care malpractice is preferred over the traditional definition for several reasons. From a risk-management perspective, its inclusiveness helps to focus the attention of health care system and organization managers, educators, and clinicians on more parameters than just professional negligence. Also, it serves to make everyone in the health care system aware of the fact that the legal system exists to protect the broadest range of rights of patients and clients.

Professional negligence, breach of contract, and intentional misconduct are all fault-based bases of liability. That is, each requires a finding of some degree of culpability on the part of the defendant–health care provider for the plaintiff to prevail. On the other hand, product liability and strict (absolute) liability for abnormally dangerous activities are non–fault-based, meaning that no culpability need be established for a finding of liability against a defendant. For these last two bases of liability, like vicarious (indirect) liability discussed later in the chapter, a judge or jury awards a verdict against a defendant as a

Two formulations for the definition of *health care malpractice*:

1. Traditional narrow definition: Professional (care-related) negligence only

2. Broad definition (trend): Any potential legal basis for imposition of liability, including the following:
   - Professional negligence
   - Breach of a patient–professional contractual promise
   - Liability for defective care-related equipment or products that injure patients or clients
   - Strict liability (absolute liability without regard for fault) for abnormally dangerous care-related professional activities
   - Intentional care-related provider misconduct conduct

matter of social policy. The operative question in such cases is this: "Between two innocent parties, who best can bear the burden of financial responsibility?"

Professional Negligence

Professional negligence by health care providers involves delivery of patient care that falls below the standards expected of ordinary reasonable practitioners of the same profession acting under the same or similar circumstances. Professional negligence involves, then, care that falls below the minimal acceptable standards for practice, or substandard care. To be professionally negligent means that the provider did or failed to do something in the course of patient examination, evaluation, intervention, or follow-up that other similarly situated health care professionals would not accept as constituting minimally acceptable care. Put still another way, professional negligence is legally actionable carelessness. Negligent patient care documentation by a provider, when it causes patient injury, constitutes legally actionable professional negligence-based health care malpractice.

Whether care is negligent is usually determined at trial by expert testimony by one or more professional peers. To qualify as an expert, such a witness must be familiar with (1) the care-related procedure in issue in the case and (2) the standard of care of the defendant–health care provider's

---

Qualifications of an Expert Witness Testifying on the Legal Standard of Care

In-depth knowledge of

1. The health care examination, evaluation, or intervention-related issue or issues involved in the lawsuit

2. The applicable standard of care, that is, what was expected of the defendant–health care provider at the time that care was rendered.

A patient suing a health care professional for malpractice must prove four elements at trial: (1) that the provider owed the patient a professional duty of care, (2) that the provider violated or breached the duty owed, (3) that the violation of the standard of care caused physical and/or mental injury to the patient, and (4) that, as a result, the patient is entitled to money "damages" in order to make the patient as whole again as possible. The standard (or burden) of proof for proving each of these required elements in civil malpractice trials is "preponderance of the evidence," which equates to "more likely than not" that the trier of fact (jury, or judge acting as fact finder when there is no jury in the case) believes that the patient–plaintiff's evidence presented at trial is more credible than that of the health professional–defendant.

discipline in the relevant geographical frame of reference at the time that care and alleged patient injury took place.

The Four Requisite Elements of Proof for a Patient–Plaintiff in a Health Care Malpractice Trial:

1. The defendant–health care provider owed the patient a special duty of due care.
2. The defendant–health care provider violated the special duty owed.
3. As a result, the patient was injured.
4. The patient is entitled to legally recognized money damages.

Ordinary Negligence Versus Professional Negligence

Many clinical situations involving patient injury do not involve professional negligence, but only ordinary or general negligence. Ordinary negligence, even when it occurs in the health care clinical setting, does not constitute health care malpractice.

A common form of ordinary or general negligence involves what is termed "premises liability." From falling on a slippery floor surface to being run into by a wheelchair or stretcher to being struck by an ambulance, ordinary premises negligence involves the kinds of careless mishaps that can occur in any physical setting—from a retail store to a college or university to a public street or sidewalk. Ordinary negligence, then, is not health care malpractice, as it is not directly care related. For that reason, with ordinary negligence, an injured patient usually needs not introduce expert testimony to attempt to show a breach of the professional standard of care because everyday situations such as slips and falls are within the common knowledge of lay jurors, who thus do not need experts to explain the mechanism of injury to them.

Professional Standard of Care

When cases do involve allegations of professional negligence, the plaintiff must usually establish the applicable standard of care and its breach by the defendant–health care provider. There are three different formulations of the standard of care in effect in various jurisdictions in the United States. Under the traditional view, health care professionals are compared with reasonably competent peers practicing in only the exact same community. This standard originally was applied to prevent prejudicing rural health care providers who lacked comparable access to the modern technology and resources available to urban-based colleagues. Modernly, this standard is no longer applicable.

The current majority rule is to compare a defendant–health care professional with reasonably competent peers practicing in either the same or similar communities. In one reported health care malpractice case, *Novey v. Kishawakee Community Health Services*, the court ruled that an occupational therapist was disqualified to testify about whether a physical therapist met or breached the standard of care because occupational therapy and physical therapy are different "schools of medicine." This case potentially has broad implications for health care professionals attempting to testify for or against health care professional–litigants of different disciplines on the litigant–professional's legal standard of care. (The extent of influence of the *Novey* decision on future cases depends on whether state or federal judges in cases outside of the state choose to adopt the decision as precedent. State court judges are not bound by case decisions reached by judges from other states, although such decisions may have precedential value.)

The trend regarding the standard of care is to apply a statewide or nationwide standard to all health professionals in any given discipline and to compare defendants charged with health care malpractice with reasonably competent peers acting under the same or similar circumstances, without regard to geographical limitations. Courts (by case law) and legislatures (by statute) are imposing this standard more and more because of standardization of education and training and because of advances in communications technology that remove the former disadvantages of rural or isolated practitioners. The standard of care for board-certified clinical specialists is currently a model for a uniform national standard of care.

Three Formulations for the Legal Standard of Care for Health Care Professionals

The three formulations for the legal standard of health care clinical practice all compare the defendant in a health care malpractice case with reasonably competent peers and ask whether such a peer would or could reasonably have acted like the defendant under the same or similar circumstances as existed in a pending lawsuit. The three formulations differ only in their geographical frame of reference.

1. Traditional rule: Compare defendant with peers from the same community

2. Modern majority rule: Compare defendant with peers from the same community or similar communities statewide or nationwide

3. Trend: Compare defendant with any and all peers statewide or nationwide who might be acting under the same or similar circumstances

Res Ipsa Loquitur: Inferences and Presumptions of Health Professional Negligence

Occasionally, a health care malpractice plaintiff will be unable, for reasons beyond the plaintiff's control, to prove that care-related injuries were caused by a breach of the duty of professional care by the defendant. For example, a comatose patient who is injured during surgery cannot testify about the cause of the injuries. Under such circumstances, courts may permit negligence to be inferred or require it to be presumed by a jury, against a health care professional–defendant, under a legal principle called *res ipsa loquitur* (Latin for "the thing [i.e., the injury] speaks for itself").

If negligence is deemed inferable, a jury is free to find negligence against the defendant or not, at its will. If, however, negligence is legally presumed, then the burden shifts to the defendant to produce sufficient evidence to rebut the presumption of negligence. For example, assume hypothetically that a comatose patient sustained a broken femur during or about the time that a defendant–registered nurse administered passive range of motion. If, under *res ipsa loquitur*, negligence is inferred, the jury deciding the case is free to disregard the inference, irrespective of whether the nurse's attorney puts forward evidence in an attempt to rebut the inference of negligence. If, however, negligence is presumed, the legal burden shifts from the plaintiff to the defendant–nurse's counsel to introduce evidence to rebut the presumption of negligence. Such rebuttal evidence on the part of the defendant might consist of testimony of a radiologist who read the patient's radiographs (called a fact, or percipient, witness) that the patient suffered from severe osteoporosis, which might have caused the plaintiff's femoral fracture.

For the doctrine of *res ipsa loquitur* to apply and relieve the plaintiff of carrying the sole legal burden of production of evidence in a case, three factors must be present. First, the plaintiff's injuries must be of the type that normally does not happen absent negligence on somebody's part. Second, the defendant–health care provider must have exercised exclusive control over the instrumentality that caused the

---

Res Ipsa Loquitur—When Negligence May Be Inferred or Presumed Without the Normal Burden of Proof by the Patient

1. The patient's injury was the kind that normally does not occur absent negligence.

2. The defendant–health care provider exercised exclusive control over the treatment or modality that caused the patient injury.

3. The patient did not contribute in any way to causing the injury.

plaintiff's injuries. Finally, the plaintiff must not have been contributorily negligent in causing the injury in issue.

One reported physical therapy malpractice case, *Greater Southeast Community Hospital Foundation v. Walker*, concerned a patient burned by a hot pack. In that case, the trial court allowed an inference of negligence under *res ipsa loquitur*. On appeal, the court reversed (disallowed) the verdict at the trial level in favor of the patient because testimony at trial had raised a question as to whether the patient had manipulated the hot pack during treatment. With such a question unresolved, it was ruled that it was improper for the trial-level judge to allow *res ipsa loquitur* because the hot pack might not have been under the therapist's exclusive control, but also under the patient's control, and the patient might have been contributorily negligent for having manipulated the hot pack.

Defenses to Health Care Malpractice Legal Actions

Two important defenses available to defendant–health care professionals, among many others, are the statute of limitations and comparative fault. The former is a procedural defense, and the latter is a substantive defense.

Statutes of Limitations

Statutes of limitations are legislatively enacted laws in effect in every state that limit the time period within which a private plaintiff in a civil case or a prosecutor in a criminal case may commence a lawsuit. There are often special rules applicable to health care malpractice; these vary from state to state. Generally, however, the "time clock" begins to run against a patient when the patient discovers or reasonably should have discovered that he or she was injured and knows the source (but not necessarily the cause) of the injury. The running of statutes of limitations may be interrupted or "tolled" by such factors as continuous treatment by a defendant–provider, infancy (under age 18), or mental incapacitation on the part of a plaintiff. Many states, however, as part of recent tort reform, have enacted statutes of repose, which set absolute time limits from the date of injury for initiating malpractice legal actions, irrespective of any factors or excuses.

One reported physical therapy case, *Myer v. Woodall*, concerned different statutes of limitations in effect in the state of the lawsuit for professional and ordinary negligence. What resulted was that the patient, who was allegedly injured while being transported to physical therapy, was held to have the right to sue the aide who transported the patient to physical therapy, but not the physical therapist or the hospital, because the professional statute of limitations had expired. The phenomenon of shortened statutes of limitations for health care malpractice actions, like statutes of repose, is a result of tort reform legislation designed to curb the number of health care malpractice legal actions.

Comparative Fault

Another major defense in health care malpractice legal actions is comparative fault. Comparative fault involves consideration by a judge or jury, not just of a health care professional–defendant's conduct, but also that of the patient–plaintiff. Under comparative fault principles, a defendant's liability may be reduced or, in a few jurisdictions precluded altogether, if the plaintiff violated the expected standard of reasonable care for his or her own safety. There are two formulations for assessing a plaintiff's fault. In contributory negligence jurisdictions, a plaintiff's case is dismissed and the plaintiff has no legal remedy if he or she was in any way contributorily negligent in causing his or her injuries—even 1% or less at fault. Because this "all-or-nothing" rule is so harsh, it has been subject to many exceptions, such as who had the "last clear chance" to prevent patient–plaintiff injury. Contributory negligence is not modernly applicable in the overwhelming majority of states.

Most states use comparative negligence as their rule when assessing a plaintiff's conduct. In most states using comparative negligence, a plaintiff may still prevail in a legal case if he or she was either (depending on the jurisdiction) less than 50% at fault or 50% or less at fault. A few comparative negligence states allow a plaintiff to recover irrespective of degree of fault. This concept is called "pure" comparative negligence. In a pure comparative negligence state, a patient who was 90% at fault for his or her own injuries and who sustained $2 million in damages might still recover $200,000 (10% of $2 million).

Vicarious Liability

Vicarious liability addresses (in addition to partnership liability) circumstances under which an employer, such as a health care organization or system, bears indirect legal and financial responsibility for the conduct of a person, such as an employee. The concept of vicarious liability dates back to ancient times and in legal circles is often referred to by its Latin name, *respondeat superior* ("let the master answer").

Employer Vicarious Liability

The basic rule of vicarious liability is that an employer is indirectly liable for the job-related conduct of an employee when the wrongdoer ("tortfeasor") is acting within the scope of his or her employment at the time the negligence occurred. Therefore, when a hospital-based health care provider is alleged to have committed professional negligence or care-related intentional misconduct such as sexual battery while treating a patient, the hospital employing the provider may be required to pay a money judgment if the provider's negligence or intentional misconduct is proven in court.

An employer's indirect responsibility for an employee's negligence does not excuse the individual provider who actually committed the negligence from financial responsibility. The tortfeasor is always personally responsible for the consequences of his or her own conduct. The concept of vicarious liability, however, gives the tort victim another party (usually with more available assets) to make a claim against or sue. When an employer is required to pay a settlement or judgment for the negligence of an employee, the employer then has the legal right to seek indemnification from the employee for this monetary outlay.

One might ask whether it is fair to impose liability on an employer who is innocent of any wrongdoing. In balancing the considerations between an innocent patient–victim and an equally innocent employer, the legal system weighs in favor of the patient. There are several good reasons for this. First, it is the employer, not the patient, who is best equipped to control the quality of care rendered by its health care providers. Second, the employer earns revenue from the official activities of its employees and contractors and should, therefore, bear responsibility for the activities that generate such revenue. Third, the employer is better able to bear the risk of financial loss through economic loss allocation (e.g., purchasing liability insurance and, to a lesser degree under managed care and cost-containment, establishing prices for health professional services) as part of the cost of doing business.

An employer may be held vicariously liable for wrongdoing by others who are not employees. In the relatively few cases addressing the issue, courts also have imposed vicarious liability on hospitals for the negligence of volunteers, equating unpaid volunteers with employees. For this reason, hospitals and clinics using the services of volunteers should carry liability insurance for volunteers' activities and include them in orientation to relevant policies and procedures, including work place safety measures.

Partnership Vicarious Liability

Another area of vicarious liability involves general partnerships, wherein each partner is considered to be the legal agent of the other partner. Absent an unambiguous express agreement to the contrary, each partner normally is vicariously liable for the other partners' negligent acts or omissions committed within the scope of activities of the partnership.

Exceptions to Vicarious Liability

Intentional Misconduct

There are several important exceptions to vicarious liability. Although an employer may be liable for employees' negligence, the employer may not be legally responsible for unforeseeable intentional misconduct committed by its employees. An example of such unforeseeable intentional misconduct in the health care setting might include the commission of sexual battery on a patient by an emergency room security guard or another patient. (Such conclusions about vicarious liability are acutely case specific and involve considerations of whether the employer undertook all available reasonable steps to ensure patient safety.)

Independent Contractors and Their Employees

Another exception to vicarious liability concerns independent contractors, including contract agency health care providers and their staffs. The legal system distinguishes employees, for whom an employer generally is legally responsible, from contractors, for whom an employer generally is not legally responsible. This distinction is based primarily on the degree of control the employer exercises over the physical details of the professional's work product.

In some cases, courts may hold employers vicariously liable even for contractors' actions under a legal theory called apparent agency. When a contract health care provider in a clinic is indistinguishable from an employee in the eyes of patients, for example, the law may treat the contract health care provider as an employee for purposes of vicarious liability. Therefore, prudent health care employers should take appropriate steps to ensure that patients know when they are being treated by contract professionals rather than by employees (e.g., by requiring contractors to wear name tags that identify their status as contract personnel and/or by posting photographs identifying employees and contract professionals in a clinic reception area).

Primary Employer Liability for Actions of Employees and Contractors

A health care organization or system may be directly or primarily liable for employees' or contractors' conduct. Such liability exists independent of any vicarious liability that may also apply. An employer is directly liable under the legal concepts of negligent selection and retention, for example, for the wrongful actions of employees or contractors whom the employer reasonably should have (1) rejected for employment, (2) carried out remediation for deficiencies for, or (3) discharged from employment.

Under law, hospitals and private clinics have certain responsibilities that they may not delegate to employees, professional medical staff, or independent contractors, under a legal concept called "corporate liability." Such responsibilities are called "nondelegable duties." Under corporate liability theories, courts have imposed various nondelegable duties on hospitals, including, among others, (1) a duty to use due care when selecting, privileging, and reprivileging physicians and surgeons and when evaluating the credentials and privileges (as applicable) of other primary health care providers; (2) a duty to ensure that premises and medical equipment are safe and adequate for patients, visitors, and staff; (3) a duty to establish patient care quality standards for their organizations and departments and divisions and to monitor and evaluate the quality of patient care on an ongoing basis; and (4) a duty to monitor continuously the competence of professional and support personnel within the facility.

Liability for Patient Abandonment

Legally actionable abandonment of a patient occurs when a health care provider improperly unilaterally terminates a professional relationship with a patient and may be classified as either professional negligence or intentional misconduct, depending on the circumstances of the abandonment of the patient. Many patient care-related activities can constitute actionable abandonment, from momentarily leaving a patient unattended to refusing to work overtime during an emergency. Although a health care provider has almost absolute discretion in electing whether to form a professional relationship with a patient, certain legal rules must be complied with to terminate an existing patient–professional relationship properly. The law imposes a special duty of care on a health care provider caring for a patient, similar to the special duty owed by an attorney to a client or a parent or guardian to a child under his or her charge.

Patient abandonment is a more salient issue because of managed care, under which considerations of cost containment may cause third-party payers to limit patient care to a set number of visits. Health care clinical professionals, not administrators or clerical personnel, are legally charged to determine the duration of patient care. Clinicians must seek appeal of administrative length-of-care decisions adverse to their patients and in contravention to their clinical judgment. Careful and appropriate documentation of justifications and rationale for such appeals (in memoranda not to be placed within patient care records) is crucial to minimize the likelihood of patient abandonment liability for clinical health care professionals.

Termination of the health care provider–patient relationship is justified when the patient makes a knowing, voluntary election to end the relationship, either unilaterally or jointly with the provider. The provider may unilaterally terminate the professional relationship with the patient when a medical condition being cared for has resolved. Unilateral termination of the relationship by the provider also may occur properly when, in a rehabilitation health professional's judgment, the patient has reached the zenith of his or her rehabilitative potential. Such a situation requires careful documentation in the patient's care record that will pass legal scrutiny should a health care malpractice action arise. Also, a health care professional must always communicate the fact that the patient has been discharged to a referring entity, any time a patient has received care pursuant to a referral.

Negligent Abandonment

If a patient claims that he or she was discharged prematurely, then the legal action that results may be a professional negligence-based health care malpractice action. As with any other health professional negligence case, the plaintiff–patient will have to prove four elements by a preponderance, or the greater weight, of evidence: that the provider owed a duty of care to the patient; that the provider violated the duty by negligently unilaterally terminating the professional relationship prematurely; that the provider's improper discharge of the patient caused harm to the patient ("causation"); and that the patient suffered legally cognizable damages, such as pain and suffering, additional medical expenses, and lost wages, that warrant the award of money damages in order to attempt to make the patient whole.

Intentional Abandonment

In contrast to negligent abandonment of a patient, a health care provider may also be charged with intentional abandonment of a patient, which carries with it more serious adverse consequences. As an intentional tort, intentional abandonment carries with it the possibility of a punitive (exemplary) damages award should the patient prevail at trial. In most cases, the defendant's professional liability insurer will not be obligated (or even permitted) to indemnify the insured if the intentional conduct is adjudged to be sufficiently egregious to justify the imposition of punitive damages against the defendant–health care provider.

Intentional abandonment might involve situations in which a patient is discharged for reasons such as failure to pay a bill, a personality conflict with a health care professional, or an insurance denial of reimbursement for further care. Under such circumstances, the provider must, at a minimum, give advance notice to the patient of the provider's intent to terminate the relationship, give the patient a reasonable amount of time to find a suitable substitute health care provider (if applicable), and assist the patient in finding a suitable substitute health care provider. Any information about the patient—examination findings, diagnosis, or intervention related information—must be communicated to the substitute care provider expeditiously. The provider transferring the patient must be sure to document in the patient's record the patient's relevant status at the time of discharge. As a risk-management measure, such a provider transferring a patient should also carefully memorialize in documentation the steps undertaken to assist the patient in finding a substitute care provider in an office memorandum, which should be retained for the period of the statute of limitations and then only disposed of under advisement of the provider's or health care organization's legal counsel.

Substitute Health Care Providers

Two special situations bear mentioning. One basis for an abandonment complaint might be that a health care provider left a patient in the care of a substitute health care provider while the original provider went on vacation, to a conference, or elsewhere on personal business. In settings in which patients contract for care with specific named clinicians, such as may occur in the private practice setting, such providers must be sure to obtain and document the patients' informed consent before transferring care to substitute health care providers. (In hospital and health maintenance organization settings, by contrast, patients do not normally contract for care with specific nonphysician health care providers, such as nurses; occupational, physical, and speech therapists; dieticians; social workers; and others—thus, the issue of abandonment during vacations and other periods of coverage does not normally arise for these providers in such settings.)

Abandonment Issues in the Limited Scope Practice Setting

Another problem concerns providers such as psychologists, social workers, occupational and physical therapists, nurse practitioners, nutrition care professionals, and other health care professionals who operate limited scope practices. Consider as an example a physical therapist specializing exclusively in the care of pediatric and adolescent patients with orthopedic or sports-related injuries. Is such a provider at liberty to refuse to treat an unrelated condition involving a current patient? The answer is probably "yes"; however, the clinician must inform the patient before forming the professional–patient relationship of the limited nature of his or her practice and gain the patient's informed consent to undergo limited scope care. Effective documentation of the patient's informed consent to limited scope care can be crucial in avoiding health care malpractice liability should a claim or lawsuit arise.

When a Health Care Professional May Be Required to "Abandon" a Patient

Certain circumstances may require a treating health care professional to disengage from caring for a patient, such as when the provider terminates his or her employment with a hospital or clinic or when a patient's third-party reimbursement for care terminates. Depending on the circumstances in each particular case, such a provider may be required to continue necessary care on a *pro bono*, or free of charge basis, even when third-party reimbursement terminates. Providers and health care organizations should always consult with their attorneys before discharging patients still in need of care under such circumstances.

Bases of Liability Other Than Professional Negligence

The vast majority of reported health care malpractice legal cases involve allegations of professional negligence by providers. This is so in large part because courts are reluctant to allow patients to sue for non–negligence-based breach of contract in the health care setting, in part because of the special status relationship between health care professionals and patients. Similarly, courts hesitate to permit patients to sue health care providers over injuries from defective products because the delivery of health care is generally viewed as the rendition of a professional service, not the sale of a product. This, however, is changing, as more and more health care professionals sell products in their clinical practices in order to generate necessary revenue in the managed-care practice environment. In such cases, courts may permit imposition of strict product liability when dangerously defectively designed or manufactured health care products injure patients, their family members, and third parties.

Few health care malpractice cases generally are premised exclusively on the issue of a lack of informed consent. Still, this area of legal responsibility is of great importance for all clinicians because every primary health care provider is legally and ethically responsible for obtaining patients' informed consent before treatment.

Other Settings and Consequences of Health Care Malpractice Actions

Criminal Proceedings for Conduct That Also Constitute Malpractice

Besides a civil malpractice lawsuit, a health professional alleged to engage in gross negligence, reckless conduct, or intentional misconduct may face criminal legal proceedings and adverse administrative actions before licensure boards and certification entities. Criminal actions, like civil malpractice lawsuits, are judicial proceedings but differ in that a state or federal prosecutor brings the criminal case against the defendant on behalf of public interests, rather than the interests of an individual victim. Because the prospective penalties are more severe, the standard of proof—beyond a reasonable doubt—is much higher than the preponderance of evidence (or greater weight of evidence) standard generally in effect in civil court.

The consequences of a finding of liability in a civil malpractice trial and a finding of guilt in a criminal trial are also different. If a civil defendant is adjudged liable, the patient–plaintiff normally is awarded compensatory money damages for expenses such as lost wages, medical expenses, pain and suffering, loss of enjoyment of life, and property losses. Normally, a civil defendant's insurer indemnifies the insured and pays off such a money judgment. In egregious cases involving reckless or intentional misconduct, a civil jury or judge may award punitive damages to a plaintiff, for which a defendant's insurer might lawfully refuse to indemnify. The penalties for a criminal defendant found guilty of a crime normally are limited to incarceration (or the threat of incarceration, i.e., probation) and a monetary fine.

Administrative and Professional Affiliation Actions

Adverse administrative actions affecting licensure and/or certification and ability to practice one's profession may be taken by state administrative licensing agencies and certification entities and, in the case of licensure, typically require a hearing to protect the constitutional due process rights of the respondent (administrative counterpart to a defendant). Private professional association actions affecting association membership may likewise result from adverse actions involving ethical infractions.

Malpractice Trial Practice and Procedures

Roles of Health Care Professionals in Malpractice Proceedings

A health care provider can take one of three roles in a civil malpractice proceeding: fact witness, expert witness, or defendant. The fact witness is probably the most familiar role. Also called an eyewitness or percipient witness, the fact witness possesses relevant first-hand knowledge about the issues and merits of a legal case important to one or both sides. A percipient witness might include a health care clinician, aide, or chaperone who carried out or observed patient care activities involving a patient–litigant. Like experts and defendants, fact witnesses may be called on to answer questions in interviews or under oath in depositions by one or both parties in a case during the pre-trial, case-building "discovery" phase of the trial process. Fact witnesses normally do not have the discretion to withhold their testimony or admissible opinions, and they normally testify subject to a subpoena or court order. Fact witnesses are normally reimbursed according to fixed (low) statutory fee schedules, rather than being allowed the opportunity to negotiate higher fees with the party calling them to testify, as are experts.

Primary nonphysician health care professionals find themselves more frequently in the role of health care malpractice defendant, as disciplines other than medicine are increasingly swept up in the malpractice litigation crisis. As a party defendant, a health care professional faces serious adverse professional and personal consequences should a verdict be rendered against him or her, including monetary loss, loss of reputation and goodwill, and adverse administrative actions at the state and federal levels. This fact is not presented with the intention to frighten health care providers but rather to familiarize them with the legal system and its processes and to make them aware of the need to seek out and obtain legal representation expeditiously whenever a potentially compensable event such as a patient injury ripens into a claim or lawsuit. It is vitally important to follow legal counsel's advice and, in particular, to refrain from talking about any potential or actual legal action against you with anyone except counsel or counsel's agents (e.g., paralegal professionals and investigators working for the health care provider's attorney). The same admonition applies to written correspondence about a pending case when you are a health care malpractice defendant. Do not send any out without legal counsel's review and concurrence.

Pretrial Proceedings

A health care provider must notify his or her facility legal department, personal insurance representative, and personal attorney (if applicable) immediately on receipt of any legal papers concerning a patient's care. When a lawsuit is filed, the first papers served normally are the "summons" (notice of lawsuit) and the "complaint" (specifying an incident allegedly causing patient injury and the amount of money damages sought). An insurer will expeditiously assign legal counsel to the case to file an "answer" to the patient–plaintiff's "pleadings."

After the complaint, answer, and other responsive papers have been exchanged and filed with the court having "jurisdiction" (control) over the case, pretrial discovery begins in earnest. The parties to the lawsuit may require each other (but not each other's witnesses) to answer formal questions called "interrogatories." The defendant–health care provider may even be called on by the plaintiff to concede liability in what is called a "request for admissions." Documents, including patient treatment records, will be requested by the patient's attorney, and other tangible evidence, such as instrument and equipment used in the course of treatment, may have to be produced for inspection by the plaintiff's expert(s).

Depositions: Procedures and Precautions

The deposition is probably the most familiar discovery device because many health care professionals have undergone deposition as witnesses or potential or actual malpractice defendants in the past. A deposition consists of sworn testimony of a party or potential party to a lawsuit, or of a fact or expert witness. It is usually taken in the office of the attorney representing the "deponent" (person being deposed) or in another seemingly informal environment. To reduce stress, try to avoid being deposed at your health care organization, where, among other things, interruptions by staff, patients, vendors, and others might affect your concentration on the legal proceedings.

Irrespective of where a deposition takes place, do not as a deponent be lulled into a false sense of security because of the apparent informality of the deposition process. A deposition is a serious legal proceeding, the consequences of which are as important as trial testimony. A court reporter transcribes every word—formal and informal—that every participant in the deposition says. The transcribed deposition may later be introduced at trial, especially to refute trial testimony as inconsistent with prior sworn testimony given at the deposition.

If health care professionals reading this section take just one piece of advice from it, it is that they should never undergo a deposition either as a witness or defendant without prior consultation with and preparation by an attorney. This does not mean that every deponent needs to have an attorney present to represent him or her at deposition. Bear in mind, however, that a health professional deponent called merely as a witness to an event one day may be named as a health care malpractice defendant the next day as a result of deposition testimony. One of the primary purposes of depositions is for attorneys for both plaintiff(s) and defendant(s) to discover relevant facts that will lead to evidence that will enable them to prevail at trial or facilitate a pretrial settlement of the case.

> Never undergo a deposition either as a witness or defendant without prior consultation with and preparation by an attorney.

Health Care Professionals as Expert Witnesses

The overwhelming majority of malpractice (and all other legal) cases are disposed of through means short of resorting to trial, principally through pretrial settlement. Should a health care malpractice case progress to trial, however, the verdict will probably turn on expert testimony. Health care professionals may qualify as experts for many purposes (e.g., as rehabilitation consultants on a patient–plaintiff's rehabilitation or vocational needs or potential); however, the principal area in which they testify as experts in malpractice proceedings is as clinical experts on whether a defendant–health care provider's treatment of a patient–plaintiff met or breached the legal standard of care.

An expert witness on the standard of care may testify for either the patient–plaintiff or for the health care provider or organization–defendant. To meet the legal standard of care and avoid being adjudged negligent, a clinical health care professional caring for a patient must exercise that special knowledge and skill characteristic of reasonably competent peers acting under the same or similar circumstances. More specifically, a health care professional must use examination, evaluative, diagnostic, prognostic, and intervention techniques and procedures that constitute at least minimally acceptable professional practice. Always bear in mind that legally acceptable care equates to minimally acceptable standards of practice, not necessarily what is optimal or even average.

Before testifying as an expert on a professional standard of care, a witness must first be qualified as legally "competent," based on expertise concerning the specific aspect of patient care at issue in the case. Oftentimes, the opponent's attorney will offer to stipulate to the qualifications of an expert witness. In such a case, the judge and jury do not have an opportunity to hear about the expert's academic background, professional publications history, or other individual attributes and achievements. Counsel proffering a witness as an expert may wish, in such situations, to seek the court's permission to enter the witness's qualifications into the record anyway. This exposure to the expert's qualifications will enhance the credibility of the expert in the eyes of the fact finder and may lead to the fact finder giving greater weight to the expert's testimony and opinions during deliberations on liability.

A very important item of documentation in support of health care malpractice litigation is the expert witness report. This document is used by plaintiff–patients and defendant–health care providers and organizations to bolster their cases. Anyone serving as a consulting expert to a party to litigation should coordinate with the employing legal counsel before reducing an oral report to writing. Written expert witness reports may be legally "discoverable" by opposing counsel, even though they are considered semiprotected "attorney work product." Ideas generated by an expert working for an attorney, however, enjoy greater protection from involuntary release under a deliberative processes exemption.

All health care professionals should consider it a civic duty to honor a request by an attorney or a court or other public agency to testify as an expert on the standard of care in a civil case or administrative legal action. If health professionals from the same discipline as a defendant under charges do not come forward and assume responsibility for so testifying, members of other disciplines may fill the void and opine on another profession's practice standards, perhaps in an incomplete or incorrect manner. Attorneys and judges in individual cases will normally seek out appropriate expert witnesses from academic and clinical settings or through referral by litigants and others in the trial process.

Potential and current expert witnesses must maintain and disseminate a fee schedule to prospective clients. The fee schedule for services must be reasonable for the market in order to be legal and ethical. Components of a fee schedule include charges for consulting, reviewing patient health records, report writing, travel time, and testifying at either deposition or trial. After an expert commits to being a testifying expert, he or she is ethically bound to live up to that commitment.

Some states have enacted tort reform legislation that affects expert witness reports. In Texas, for example, since 2004, parties to health care malpractice litigation (patient–plaintiffs and health care provider–defendants) must file expert witness reports (including experts' curricula vitae) within 120 days after filing a health care malpractice claim with the other side. The party receiving that report then has only 21 days to challenge the adequacy of the report. These measures help prevent frivolous legal actions from proceeding to depositions and trial.

With tens of millions of civil lawsuits filed or pending in state and federal courts in the United States, far ahead of all other civilized nations combined, there clearly is a serious litigation crisis in the United States. In large and relatively litigious states, civil cases, including health care malpractice lawsuits, can take many years to come to trial.

The National Practitioner Data Bank

Since September 1990, whenever money (in any sum) is paid to a patient–plaintiff or his or her representative, either in settlement or by way of a court judgment in a health care malpractice case, information about the responsible health care provider must be forwarded to the Department of Health and Human Services for inclusion in the National Practitioner Data Bank. This data bank was established pursuant to the Health Care Quality Improvement Act of 1986.

Another important purpose of the data bank is to compile data concerning adverse licensure and credentialing actions, as well as expulsion from professional associations, involving licensed health care providers. Together, malpractice payment reporting and adverse actions reporting are intended to create a record that follows licensed health care professionals included in the data bank wherever in the United States they might seek employment.

Employers of licensed health care professionals are required under the statute to query the data bank regarding new employees and at regular intervals thereafter. The information is deemed strictly confidential and normally is not "discoverable" by patients or their attorneys. Data bank information is not available to the general public. As an exception to the nondisclosure provision, if a health care employer fails to query the data bank about a provider upon employment, a patient–plaintiff's attorney may petition for, and be granted, access to that provider's data bank information.

Although the data bank records credentialing and malpractice payment information on all licensed health care providers, it only records licensure information on physicians and dentists. Any licensed health care provider may self-query the data bank for a nominal fee at www.npdb-hipdb.com.

Chapter Exercise 4

If you are already a licensed health care professional, query the National Practitioner Data Bank for a copy of your own record (for a nominal fee) at www.npdb-hipdb.hrsa.gov.

Tort Reform Measures

The federal government and most state legislatures have undertaken, since the advent of the litigation and health care malpractice crises, reforms focused on patient care documentation. Many of these public entities have also undertaken measures labeled as "tort reform" to decrease the number of civil lawsuits. Some of these reform measures include the following:

1. Enacting and, after substantial delay, implementing HIPAA (the federal Health Insurance Portability and Accountability Act of 1996).

2. Limiting time periods for validity of undated patient health information release authorizations, as initiated by Texas in 1998.

3. Requiring that health care malpractice plaintiffs undergo administrative hearings on the merits of their cases before proceeding to trial.

4. Capping maximum noneconomic money damages for pain and suffering and loss of enjoyment of life. (This reform has been introduced on seven occasions since 1995 in Congress, but as of May 2006, no comprehensive federal tort reform statute has been enacted by both the Senate and House. In fact, on May 8, 2006, the Senate took health care malpractice reform off the agenda for the year. The most recent version of the federal bill would have limited payments to successful malpractice plaintiffs for pain and suffering to $250,000. The nonpartisan Congressional Budget Office predicts that federal limits on health care malpractice payments would reduce the percentage of aggregate health care expenditures attributable to malpractice from 2% to 1.5%.)

5. Limiting attorney contingent fees (contingent fees are based on percentages of recovery fees bargained for between attorneys and clients). California was the first state to do this in 1975.

6. Reforming joint and several liability to prevent one defendant from being required to pay an entire judgment when that defendant is only partially responsible for a plaintiff's injuries.

7. Setting absolute time limits—based on the date of injury or manufacture of a product—within which legal action must be commenced (called statutes of repose).

8. Relaxing the collateral source rule, under which juries are prevented from learning of a plaintiff's collateral sources of compensation for injuries, including insurance coverage or partial payments by other defendants.

9. Penalizing attorneys and their clients for initiating lawsuits deemed to be frivolous, especially in the federal courts.

10. Withholding from plaintiffs (and depositing in state treasuries) a percentage of any "punitive" (punishment) damages awarded to them by juries in product liability actions.

A Framework for Professional Ethical Decision Making

All health care professionals need to have in place a framework for identifying and resolving ethical problems, issues, and dilemmas that arise in practice. This is true irrespective of one's discipline and practice setting.

An ethics framework is a working model of the processes used to identify and resolve practice-related problems. It is augmented by substantive reference and decisional inputs, such as discipline-specific codes of ethics, practice acts, protocols and guidelines, and legal inputs, including fact sheets from institution or system attorneys, conference notes, textbooks, and journal articles. When faced with an ethical issue, one can always seek outside advice from professional colleagues in the work place, institutional ethics committees, association attorneys, and individual legal counsel, among possible others. In the end, however, each health care professional must personally resolve the ethical practice problems, issues, and dilemmas that he or she encounters and bear responsibility for such decisions. This is the essence of being a professional.

The ethics model that I have used and refined since the late 1960s is a systems model. I call it the systems model for health professional ethical decision making. It was first published *Professional Ethics: A Guide for Rehabilitation*

> Each health care professional must personally resolve the ethical practice problems, issues, and dilemmas that he or she encounters and bear responsibility for decisions made. This is the essence of being a professional.

Professionals (Mosby 1998). The model includes four simple steps: identification of a problem, issue, or dilemma; stating facts and unknowns and making relevant assumptions; delineating viable options for resolution and implementing the optimal one; and monitoring implementation of an option for efficacy and making any necessary modifications to the chosen course of action. It is the monitoring feedback mechanism of this model that is characteristic of the systems approach.

My model is only one of many in the health professional literature that may be adapted for health professionals' use in the field. In the end, the best model for each professional is one that is carefully contemplated and personally developed and refined. Such a model may take years of experience to come to fruition.

QUESTIONS AND CASES FOR STUDY

1. In your opinion, should the nations of the world retain or discard diplomatic immunity? Make a list of five reasons favoring each of the two positions.

2. Compare and contrast any licensed health care discipline's professional association code of ethics and its state practice act. How are the two documents similar? How do they differ (if at all)?

3. A is an orthopedic patient with chronic cervical pain, being seen for the first time by B, an outpatient physical therapist. No documentation except the prescription, properly signed by the referring physician, is present with the patient at the initial visit. During the course of examination, B asks A if any x-rays had been taken. A replies "yes," and adds, "I think the doctor said they were okay." Should B proceed with mechanical traction treatment based on the examination findings and A's self-report about her x-rays?

4. In your opinion, should Congress enact federal health care malpractice reform and limit patient injury awards to $250,000? Make a list of 10 expected consequences of such reform. Who pays for continuing care for these patient–plaintiffs after the $250,000 awards are expended?

5. Adapt your personal model for health professional ethical decision making to a flow diagram format. If you are in a classroom setting, share students' and the professor's models. What do they have in common? Synthesize variables into a single model.

REFERENCES, READINGS, AND RESOURCES

1. Americans with Disabilities Act, 42 U.S.C. 12101–12213.

2. Brody JA. Just what the doctor ordered? Not exactly. *New York Times.* May 9, 2006, D6.

3. Brown D. *The Da Vinci Code.* New York: Doubleday, 2003.

4. Eickhoff J. Exercise equipment injuries: Who's at fault? *ACSM's Health & Fitness Journal.* 2002;6:27–30.

5. Furrow B, et al. *Health Law: Cases, Materials and Problems,* 5th ed. St. Paul, MN: West Publishing Co., 2004.

6. *Greater Southeast Community Hosp. Found. v. Walker.* 313 A.2d 105 (D.C. 1973).

7. *Griswold v. Connecticut.* 381 U.S. 479 (1965).

8. Hanks GC, Polinger-Hymen R. Redefining the battlefield: Expert reports in medical malpractice litigation after HB4. *Texas Bar Journal.* 2004; Dec.:936–944.

9. Kearney KA, McCord FL. Hospital management faces new liabilities. *Health Law.* 1992; Fall:1–6.

10. Keeton WP. *Prosser and Keeton on Torts,* 5th ed. St. Paul, MN: West Law Publishers, Inc., 1984.

11. Health Insurance Portability and Accountability Act of 1996, 42 U.S.C. 1320.

12. Leitner DL. *Managed Care Liability.* Chicago: American Bar Association (Tort and Insurance Practice Section), 1996.

13. *Myer v. Woodall.* 592 P.2d 1343 (Colo. Ct. App. 1979).

14. *Novey v. Kishawaukee Community Health Serv.* 531 N.E.2d 427 (Ill. App. Cf. 4989).

15. Occupational Safety and Health Act, 29 U.S.C. 651–678.

16. *Roe v. Wade.* 410 U.S. 113 (1973).

17. Scott RW. *Legal Aspects of Documenting Patient Care for Rehabilitation Professionals,* 3rd ed. Sudbury, MA: Jones and Bartlett, 2006.

18. Scott RW. Supporting professional development: Understanding the interplay between health law and professional ethics. *Journal of Physical Therapy Education.* 2000;14(3):17–19.

19. Scott RW. *Health Care Malpractice: A Primer on Legal Issues,* 2nd ed. New York: McGraw-Hill, Inc., 1999.

20. Scott RW. *Professional Ethics: A Guide for Rehabilitation Professionals.* St. Louis: Mosby, Inc., 1998.

21. Stolberg SG. Senate rejects award limits in malpractice. *New York Times.* May 9, 2006, A18.

22. www.healthgrades.com

23. www.iom.edu [Institute of Medicine]

24. www.juryverdictresearch.com

25. www.npdb-hipdb.hrsa.gov [National Practitioner Data Bank]

Chapter 4

Personal and Professional Self-Appraisal and Management

ABSTRACT

Do you have what it takes to prepare for, become, develop professionally, and remain a health care professional? Are you prepared to take on all that may be required in order to become one? Through the processes of introspection and completing selected self-assessment instruments, you can definitively answer these questions. Every health care professional—prospective and practicing—must be ready to subordinate personal interests, and the interests of others, in favor of those of patients and clients under care. A health professional is a fiduciary, charged by law, ethics, and custom to put patients' interests first. One of the most important attributes of a fiduciary is respect for patient autonomy and privacy. Such respect engenders confidence that permits free communication between health professionals and patients. From respect for patient advance directives (end-of-life decisional instruments) to informed consent to patient personal health information privacy, the health professional fiduciary bears formidable responsibilities toward patients under care.

KEY WORDS AND PHRASES

- Advance directives
- Affective domain
- Cognitive domain
- Deficiency needs
- Fiduciary
- Growth needs
- Hierarchy of human needs
- HIPAA

- Informational interview
- Informed consent
- Introspection
- Patient Self-Determination Act
- Privacy
- Protected health information
- Psychomotor domain

- Self-actualization
- Self-appraisal
- Self-determination
- Standard operating procedure
- Surrogate decision maker
- Values survey

OBJECTIVES

1. Assess your interest in selected health care professions through self-assessment and informational interviews.
2. Always present a professional demeanor as a health care professional.
3. Understand and execute the complex role of fiduciary for patients under your care and their significant others.
4. Respect and safeguard patient private health information from unauthorized and unnecessary disclosures.
5. Develop and use a process for universally obtaining patient (or surrogate decision maker) informed consent to health care services.

Self-Assessment

So you want to become a health professional? You have already carefully researched the myriad of health care disciplines and their specialties and have selected one for your potential career goal. You may have spoken with guidance counselors in your high school or college, or perhaps you have spoken with a career consultant. Maybe you have visited the work place of one or more professionals in your selected field to conduct informational interviews to learn more about the profession. You are probably soon ready to (or already have in process) making applications for entry into an entry-level professional education program.

> An informational interview with a health professional is a great way to explore and learn more about any given health profession.

Now is the time to carry out serious self-assessment before proceeding. Self-assessment involves the processes by which one looks inward to evaluate parameters such as one's attitudes, interests, personality traits, cognitive and psychomotor skills sets, and values. This process of introspection helps you guide your search for a career and employment by helping you to determine where (career-wise, practice setting-wise, and geographically) you will be happiest and most productive—that is, the "best fit."

> Self-assessment is the process by which one looks inward to evaluate parameters such as one's attitudes, interests, personality traits, cognitive and psychomotor skills sets, and values.

Abraham Maslow established a hierarchy of human needs, which all people strive to satisfy. They are, in order from lowest to highest: physiological needs, safety and security needs, socialization needs, self-determination, and self-actualization. Physiological needs include food, water, shelter, and basic transportation. Safety and security needs seem more important now, after 9-11. According to Solomon and King, the American work place has become less safe over the past several decades. In fact, work place violence is the third leading cause of occupational deaths. Since 1980, an average of 750 people per year have been victims of work place homicides. Most of these homicides (75%) are committed with firearms.

Socialization or group dynamics constitutes the highest order deficiency need. People are naturally gregarious and most thrive in work environments with other people present. Elton Mayo, a Harvard sociologist, found in his famous Hawthorne experiment in the 1920s that workers with a modicum of collective autonomy over their work and workspace were more productive and had higher morale than those lacking such control.

The two highest personal needs—self-determination and self-actualization—are labeled growth needs. Through their fulfillment, individuals become Renaissance people. Self-determination involves the right of choice over one's actions and involves the highest level of reflective thinking. It encompasses professional autonomy and the right to be creative and innovative in the work place. Self-actualization entails the full utilization of one's talents and potential for the good of humankind. When one achieves self-actualization, one has truly "arrived."

In your professional growth path, always aspire to fulfill the two highest order growth needs—self-determination (the hallmark of a professional) and self-actualization (the hallmark of a happy, complete individual). Achievement of these two goals is obtainable for every professional, irrespective of his or her occupational discipline.

A large number of self-assessment resource tools and instruments are available in print and online. Self-assessment instruments may be either self-directed and self-scoring or may require the interpretive assistance of trained professionals. Many are available free of charge.

The following are representative resources for selected self-assessment areas. One of the most widely used general career guides is the book *What Color Is Your Parachute?* (Bolles RN, Berkeley, CA: Ten Speed Press, current edition). Another recommended Internet site, geared to teens seeking careers, is Kidzonline.org.

Perhaps the most widely used personality indices are the Minnesota Multiphasic Personality Inventory-2 (MMPI-2) and the Myers-Briggs (Personality) Type Indicator (MBTI). The former instrument is mainly used by psychologists to identify psychological impairments and the latter by human resource professionals to evaluate employees in work settings. The latter is an assessment that can help identify respondents as persons who obtain their energy internally or externally, prefer facts or ideas as decisional inputs, are logical or values oriented, and are relatively organized or flexible. I have taken this personality instrument at three very disparate times in my career and have consistently scored the same way each time. I find it to be highly reliable and valid. To learn more about Myers-Briggs, visit www.myersbriggs.org.

Perhaps the best way to self-assess cognitive and psychomotor skill sets required for various health career fields is to examine the requisites listed in the Nature of the Work and Working Conditions sections for your chosen discipline(s) in the Bureau of Labor Statistics' Occupational Outlook Handbook. After you peruse the physical and mental qualifications for your chosen field(s), assess whether you "have what it takes" to succeed in the selected field(s).

Many values self-assessment instruments are available online to prospective career seekers. One of the best in my opinion is the Ohio Learning Network's Career Values Survey, available at www.oln.org.

Consider first the following basic health careers self-assessment instrument:

Chapter Exercise 1

Answer the following 10 questions honestly and carefully and reflect on your written responses. Save your responses and revisit them 10, 25, and 50 years from now.

1. Why do you want to become a health care professional?
2. What discipline/specialty interests you most? Why?
3. Have you taken time to explore your field of interest? If so, what are your early impressions about this career field?
4. Which of your personal strengths make you particularly suited for a health professions career?
5. Name three areas in which you could benefit from personal development or improvement?
6. Do you like more to work alone or with people?
7. Do you work well under pressure? How well do you function under high pressure?

8. Which is more important to you—wealth accumulation or service to others?
9. Do you work well with your hands? Do you work well with your mind? Both equally well?
10. How will you finance your education and balance the work, school, and personal time components of your life?
11. Do you believe that people have a duty to give something back to society and its people for the good things they receive?
12. What major contribution(s) do you hope to make to society through your career?

Focus on Fiduciaries and Respect for Patient Privacy

Being a True Fiduciary: Respecting Patient Autonomy and Privacy Rights

Health care professionals are fiduciaries to the patients under their care and to their legally appointed surrogate decision makers and agents acting under durable powers of attorney for health care decision making. As fiduciaries, they are charged by law and ethics to put patients' interests above all others, including their own. One of the key fiduciary duties owed to patients by health care professionals at all levels is the duty to safeguard patient privacy. Patients find themselves as a matter of course exposed and vulnerable to excessive scrutiny and exploitation by others. From professional and support staff to clerical and administrative professionals to third-party payers to quality management reviewers, many private aspects of patients' lives that otherwise would not be are open to public scrutiny.

Basic Privacy Principles

There is both a common law right of privacy, as established in judge-made case law, and a constitutional right of privacy. The common law right of privacy protects individuals, such as patients, from unreasonable violations of their personal privacy by other persons or entities. The implied federal constitutional right of privacy protects individuals' privacy from unwarranted invasion by governmental entities and agents.

After 9-11, compelling national security interests have seriously undermined considerations of privacy. Everything from international telephone calls to domestic call logs to Internet servers has been open to governmental scrutiny.

The recent diminution in importance for privacy has carried over to health care as well. Many or most primary health care professionals do not believe that patients have the right to absolutely control what information is in their health records. This particularly applies to results of evaluative tests and measurements. Results of genetic testing discovered by insurers in patients' health records may result in insurance denials and adverse employment consequences, despite an inconsistent patchwork of genetic antidiscrimination laws across the 50 states. Federal genetic antidiscrimination laws apply to only group, not individual, insurance policies.

Chapter Exercise 2

Consider the following case:

Patient X carries her health record with her from Dr. Y's clinic. After perusing the pages, she sees a reference to her positive HIV status in a physical examination report. X removes that page from her record and returns the incomplete record on her next visit. Did X have the right to remove this information from her record?

(For a psychiatrist's perspective on this subject, see Klitzman R. The Quest for Privacy Can Make Us Thieves. *New York Times,* May 9, 2006, A22.)

Patient Advance Directives

The Patient Self-Determination Act, signed into law by former President Bush in November 1990, codifies a patient's common law right to control health care decisions—both routine and extraordinary. When it became effective on December 1, 1991, the act bound hospitals, health maintenance organizations, long-term care facilities, hospices, and other health care entities participating in Medicare and Medicaid to its provisions.

The fundamental purpose of the act is to ensure that providers and health care organizations provide patient education about informed consent and the right of patients to make advance directives. *Advance directives* include legal instruments such as the living will, durable power of attorney for health care decision making, out-of-facility do-not-resuscitate order, and declaration for mental health treatment, which memorialize patient desires concerning life-sustaining measures to be taken and decision making should the patient subsequently become legally incapacitated.

A key concept underlying the act is respect for a patient's right to give informed consent to health-related examination and intervention. Although the act does not create any new substantive patient rights, it does impose burdensome procedural obligations on health care organizations and providers covered by the law. Among other mandates, the act requires a covered health care provider or facility to

(1) (A) Provide written information [to patients] concerning

      (i) an individual's rights under state law (whether statutory or as recognized by the courts of the state) to make decisions concerning . . . medical care, including the right to accept or refuse medical or surgical treatment and the right to formulate advance directives

      (ii) the written policies of the provider or organization respecting the implementation of such rights

  (B) Document in the individual's medical record whether the individual has executed an advance directive

(2) The written information described in paragraph (1)(A) shall be provided to an adult individual:

  (A) in the case of a hospital, at the time of the individual's admission as an inpatient

  (B) In the case of a skilled nursing facility, at the time of the individual's admission as a resident

  (C) In the case of a home health agency, in advance of the individual coming under the care of the agency

Before any substantive care is undertaken, then, in any patient care setting, a patient must receive written information about the right to make informed decisions regarding examination and intervention and the right (consistent with state law) to make advance directives regarding future care in the event of the patient's incapacitation. Also, a covered health care facility must provide the patient with a written copy of the facility's policy on implementing the requirements of the act.

In addition to its disclosure obligations discussed previously, a health care organization covered by the act has documentation responsibilities as well. The facility must annotate in a patient's care record whether the patient has signed an advance directive regarding future care.

The three relevant questions that a facility's staff must ask of patients are as follows:

1. Do you have any advance directives? If so, what kind?
2. Do you have a copy of your directive(s)?
3. Have there been any changes to your directives? If so, what are they, and do you have documentation of the changes?

Larsen and Eaton carried out an exhaustive study of the act and reported that the act has been relatively unsuccessful in safeguarding the rights of patients to make and have enforced advance directives concerning health care. The reasons cited for the lack of success of the act include the following:

- Lack of individual awareness on the part of primary health care professionals of the existence of the act
- Reluctance on the part of patients and long-term care facility residents to execute advance directives
- Recalcitrance on the part of health care providers and organizations to honor valid advance patient directives, in part because they substitute their own values for those of patients or they fear liability exposure

Informed Consent

The following elements normally must be disclosed to the patient before examination or intervention; then patient (or surrogate) questions must be actively solicited by the primary health care provider, and any questions that the patient has must be satisfactorily answered by that provider in order to meet the legal requirements for patient informed consent. The exact requirements for informed consent vary from state to state, however. This list that follows does not necessarily represent the law of any particular state. (See your facility or personal attorney for specific advice.)

> As primary health care providers, always bear in mind that any health-related intervention is only a recommended intervention (even if prescribed or ordered by another health care professional) unless and until a patient with legal and mental capacity agrees to it.

Patient informed consent to examination involves disclosure and discussion of the patient's medical or other prior relevant diagnosis and the parameters of the intended examination. For a patient's consent to substantive intervention to be legally sufficient, or "informed," the primary health care provider must relate the following elements to the patient in lay person's language at the level of patient understanding:

1. A description of the patient's health problem (diagnosis or evaluative findings) and the recommended intervention.

2. Material risks, if any, associated with the recommended intervention. Material risks include important "decisional" risks (including foreseeable complications associated with the recommended intervention) or precautions that would cause an ordinary, reasonable patient to think carefully when deciding whether to undergo or reject the recommended intervention.

3. Reasonable alternatives, if any, to the proposed intervention (i.e., other effective potential interventions that would be acceptable substitutes

under legal standards of practice). The provider must be sure to include discussion of the relative risks and benefits of alternative interventions.

4. Expected benefits or goals and prognosis associated with the recommended intervention.

Providers should memorize these elements and routinely cover each of them with every patient. After the applicable disclosure elements are imparted to a patient, the health care provider must solicit patient questions and answer them to the patient's satisfaction before proceeding on to either examination or intervention.

When the English language is not a patient's primary language (or that of the surrogate decision maker for patients lacking mental capacity), the provider must use the services of an interpreter to ensure patient comprehension of the informed consent disclosure elements. Careful documentation is recommended whenever an interpreter is employed during these processes. An example of documenting the services of an interpreter during informed consent disclosure appears here.

Example of Informed Consent Documentation Involving an Interpreter for the Patient

ABC General Hospital
Rehabilitation Center, Physical Therapy Section
May 23, 200x / 1600

S: 42 y o F, dx multiple sclerosis, wheelchair-bound, referred for "evaluation, facilitative range of motion, and progressive exercise and ambulation, to tolerance." Pt. is Spanish-speaking; Mrs. Gonzales, Red Cross volunteer, acted as interpreter.

O: . . .

A: . . .

P: Begin AAROM today; standing at parallel bars, to tolerance. I obtained informed consent from the pt. in Spanish through Mrs. Gonzales, interpreter. Pt. verbalizes understanding of her diagnosis and my examination findings; the recommended intervention as outlined in Dr. Doe's order; the risks of muscle soreness, fatigue, and the slight risk of joint subluxation associated with exercise; and information about the alternative options of bedrest and limited activity in her wheelchair. I asked for her questions, through Mrs. Gonzales. She wanted to know how long sessions lasted; I told her 45 min to 1 hr. each, but only to her tolerance. She verbalized satisfaction with the program as outlined and agreed to try it.

G: . . .

Reggie Hausenfus, PT, #07165733

Checklist Disclosure Elements for Patient Informed Consent to Intervention:

- Examination and evaluative findings; diagnosis (or diagnoses)
- Description of the recommended intervention(s)
- Material (decisional) risks of possible harm or foreseeable complications associated with the recommended intervention(s)
- Expected benefits (goals) and prognosis
- Reasonable alternatives to the recommended intervention, including relative risks, benefits, and prognosis associated with reasonable alternative interventions (or no intervention)
- Solicit and satisfactorily answer patient question

HIPAA

HIPAA (the Health Insurance Portability and Accountability Act of 1996), is a federal law that is designed to ensure portability of employee health benefits when employees change jobs and a system for maximizing patient protected health information privacy. HIPAA's provisions related to protected health information (PHI) privacy include the Privacy and Security Rules and the Electronic Data Transmission Standards.

The Privacy Rule, effective since April 14, 2003, is designed to prevent unauthorized and unwarranted disclosure of patient PHI. Health care systems, plans, providers, and clearinghouses that conduct financial transactions electronically must be committed to compliance with the letter and spirit of HIPAA in receiving, processing, storing, transmitting, and otherwise handling patient/client PHI.

HIPAA's privacy standards represent the first comprehensive federal guidelines for protection of PHI. Supplemental guidance and protections are found in state and local case law, statutes, and administrative rules and regulations. Protection extends to any individually identifiable health information, maintained or transmitted in any medium, held by any covered entity or business associate of a covered entity.

Covered entities must obtain adequate contractual assurances from business associates that the latter will appropriately safeguard patient PHI that comes to them. Examples of activities that may be conducted by business associates include benefit management, billing, claims processing, data analysis, quality-improvement management, practice management, and utilization review. If a business associate is found to have violated HIPAA, the covered entity must first attempt to "cure" (correct) the breach (violation) (of contract) and, if unsuccessful, terminate the contract with the noncompliant business associate and report the matter to the Secretary of the Department of Health and Human Services for follow-on administrative action.

Each employee, contractor, and consultant is a fiduciary, owing a personal duty to patients to take all reasonable steps pursuant to HIPAA to safeguard their PHI. All employees and other providers must receive HIPAA training during initial orientation and periodically thereafter to update their knowledge base about HIPAA.

> Providers and entities covered by HIPAA must exercise reasonable caution under all circumstances to disclose only the minimum necessary amount of PHI in order to comply with their legal duties owed to patients and others.

On the first visit to any covered provider, all patients must be made aware of the facility's HIPAA Privacy Policy. Direct care providers must issue a Patient Notice of Privacy Practices to all patients at first contact and make a good-faith attempt to obtain patients' written acknowledgment of receipt of the document. In addition, providers must post their entire Patient Notice of Privacy Practices in their facility in a prominent location for patients to see. Exemplars of HIPAA Patient Notice of Privacy Practices documents in English and Spanish appear at Appendices C and D.

Normally, a covered entity (any provider filing reimbursement claims electronically) may use and disclose a patient's PHI for purposes of treatment, payment for services, and internal health care operations of the business, without the patient's authorization or consent. These disclosures are called "routine uses."

Regarding patient informed consent for routine uses of PHI, providers are required only to make a good-faith effort to obtain patient/client informed consent for treatment, payment, and healthcare operations. Covered entities have wide discretion to design processes that mesh with their individual practices. Patients/clients have the right to request restrictions on the use or disclosure of their protected health information, but covered entities are not required to agree to such restrictions.

There are three general classifications of PHI disclosures under HIPAA. They are permissive and mandatory (both without patient authorization or consent) and authorized. Permissive disclosures include those necessary for treatment, payment, and operations. This includes, among other possibilities, communication between and among treatment team members, determination of coverage for health services, and peer/utilization review activities.

Required disclosures are those made pursuant to legal mandates, such as a court order or state reporting statutes (for suspected abuse; communicable diseases, including sexually transmitted diseases; and gunshot wounds). Authorized disclosures encompass broad disclosure authority pursuant to valid written and signed patient authorization.

Regarding minors' PHI, the Privacy Rule generally allows a parent to have access to the medical records about his or her child, as his or her minor child's personal representative when such access is not inconsistent with state or other laws. There are three situations when the parent would not be the minor's personal representative under the Privacy Rule. These exceptions are (1) when the minor is the one who consents to care and the consent of the parent is not required under state or other applicable law (e.g., when the minor is emancipated); (2) when the minor obtains care at the direction of a court or a person appointed by the court; and (3) when, and to the extent that, the parent agrees that the minor and the health care provider may have a confidential relationship. Even in these exceptional situations, however, the parent may have access to the health record of the minor related to this treatment when state or other applicable law requires or permits such parental access.

The following are suggested standard operating procedures for clinics that are covered entities under HIPAA's Privacy Rule. This list is not intended to be comprehensive. In addition to appointing and adequately training a clinic privacy officer, the staffs of covered entities should brainstorm on lists of standard operating procedures to be implemented for their individual practices.

Suggested Standard Operating Procedures Pursuant to HIPAA's Privacy Rule

1. Staff will not allow patient records to be placed or to remain in open (public) view.

2. Staff will not discuss patient PHI within the hearing/perceptive range of third parties not involved in the patient's care.

3. Patients and other nonemployees/contractors/consultants are not permitted access to the patient records room.

4. Except where authorized, permitted, or required by law, PHI disclosures require HIPAA-compliant written patient/client authorizations and written requests by requestors for information.

5. Patient records may not be removed from the facility, except for transit to and from secure storage, or otherwise as authorized, permitted, or required by law.

6. Written requests by patients for their health records will be expeditiously honored.

7. Patient/client records may be placed in chart holders for clinic providers, provided that the following reasonable and appropriate measures are taken to protect the patient's privacy: limiting access to patient care areas and escorting nonemployees in the area, ensuring that the areas are supervised, and placing patient/client charts in chart holders with the front cover facing the wall rather than having protected health information about the patient visible to anyone who walks by.

8. Providers may leave phone messages for patients on their answering machines. Limit the amount of information disclosed on the answering machine to clinic name and number and any other information necessary to confirm an appointment, asking the individual to call back. It is permissible to leave a similar message with a family member or other person who answers the phone when the patient is not home.

9. The clinic is required to give the notice of its privacy policy to every individual receiving treatment no later than the date of first service delivery and to make a good-faith effort to obtain the individual's written acknowledgment of receipt of the notice.

10. The clinic is required to give the notice of its privacy policy to every individual receiving treatment no later than the date of first service delivery and to make a good-faith effort to obtain the individual's written acknowledgment of receipt of the notice. The clinic also must post its entire privacy policy in the facility in a clear and prominent location where individuals are likely to see it, as well as make the notice available to those who ask for a copy. Copies of the clinic privacy notice are maintained in English and Spanish.

Providers covered by HIPAA may still use sign-in sheets for patients and call out their names in waiting rooms as long as PHI is not disclosed in these processes. Seeing someone in a waiting room and hearing one's name called constitute "incidental" disclosures that do not violate HIPAA, according to the Department of Health and Human Services. A sign-in sheet may not, however, list patients' diagnoses.

Providers may also transmit patient health records to other providers without patient authorization or consent, if the gaining providers are treating the patient for the same condition as the sending provider. This includes transfer of an entire patient health record (including documentation created by other providers), if reasonably necessary for treatment.

Providers are not normally required to document a "disclosure history" unless patient authorization is required for disclosure; however, it would be prudent risk management to create and maintain such a history. What is required is that covered providers and entities exercise reasonable caution under all circumstances to disclose only the minimum necessary amount of PHI in order to comply with their legal duties owed to patients and others.

The HIPAA Privacy Rule does not apply to entities that are workers' compensation insurers, administrative agencies, or employers, except to the extent that they may otherwise be covered entities. These entities need access to the health information of individuals who are injured on the job or who have a work-related illness to process and adjudicate claims and to coordinate care under workers' compensation systems. Generally, this health information is obtained from health care providers who are covered by the Privacy Rule.

The Privacy Rule recognizes the legitimate need of insurers and other entities involved in the workers' compensation systems to have access to individuals' health information as authorized by state or other laws. Because of the significant variability among such laws, the Privacy Rule permits disclosures of health information for workers' compensation purposes in a number of different ways.

1. Disclosures without individual authorization. The Privacy Rule permits covered entities to disclose protected health information to workers' compensation insurers, state administrators, employers, and other persons or entities involved in workers' compensation systems, without the individual's authorization.

   a. As authorized by and to the extent necessary to comply with laws relating to workers' compensation or similar programs established by law that provide benefits for work-related injuries or illness without regard to fault. This includes programs established by the Black Lung Benefits Act, the Federal Employees' Compensation Act, the Longshore and Harbor Workers' Compensation Act, and the Energy Employees' Occupational Illness Compensation Program Act. See 45 CFR 164.512(l).

   b. To the extent the disclosure is required by State or other law. The disclosure must comply with and be limited to what the law requires. See 45 CFR 164.512(a).

   c. For purposes of obtaining payment for any health care provided to the injured or ill worker. See 45 CFR 164.502(a)(1)(ii) and the definition of "payment" at 45 CFR 164.501.

2. Disclosures with individual authorization. In addition, covered entities may disclose protected health information to workers' compensation insurers and others involved in workers' compensation systems where the individual has provided his or her authorization for the

release of the information to the entity. The authorization must contain the elements and otherwise meet the requirements specified at 45 CFR 164.508.

3. Minimum necessary. Consistent with HIPAA's Privacy Rule main theme, covered entities are required reasonably to limit the amount of protected health information disclosed under 45 CFR 164.512(l) to the minimum necessary to accomplish the workers' compensation purpose. Under this requirement, protected health information may be shared for such purposes to the full extent authorized by state or other law. In addition, covered entities are required reasonably to limit the amount of protected health information disclosed for payment purposes to the minimum necessary. Covered entities are permitted to disclose the amount and types of protected health information that are necessary to obtain payment for health care provided to an injured or ill worker. Where a covered entity routinely makes disclosures for workers' compensation purposes under 45 CFR 164.512(l) or for payment purposes, the covered entity may develop standard protocols as part of its minimum necessary policies and procedures that address the type and amount of protected health information to be disclosed for such purposes. Where protected health information is requested by a state workers' compensation or other public official, covered entities are permitted to rely reasonably on the official's representations that the information requested is the minimum necessary for the intended purpose. See 45 CFR 164.514(d)(3)(iii)(A). Covered entities are not required to make a minimum necessary determination when disclosing protected health information as required by state or other law or pursuant to the individual's authorization. See 45 CFR 164.502(b).

HIPAA-related patient complaints should first be directed to an organization's HIPAA privacy officer. A complaint may also be filed with the Office of Civil Rights, U.S. Department of Health and Human Services (DHHS).

DHHS requires the following in a written complaint:

1. Complainant's full name and residential and e-mail addresses and home and work phone numbers
2. Name, address, and phone number of entity violating complainant's PHI
3. Description of the PHI violation
4. Complainant's signature and date
5. Necessary reasonable accommodations, as applicable

An alleged PHI violator is prohibited from taking retaliatory action against a complainant. Potential sanctions for HIPAA Privacy Rule violations include civil and criminal penalties. Civil penalties of between $100 and $25,000 per violation are enforced by the Office of Civil Rights, DHHS. Criminal sanctions of 1 to 10 years of imprisonment and $50,000 to $250,000 fines are enforced by the Department of Justice.

QUESTIONS AND CASES FOR STUDY

1. Self-assess your interest in selected health care professions by perusing the Bureau of Labor Statistics' Occupational Outlook Handbook at www.bls.gov/oco.

2. Access the website www.TipsforSuccess.org. Review the self-assessment tool entitled "Are You Professional?" Rate your own professionalism on a 0–10 scale.

3. What should be the consequences if a patient removes data from her or his health record without authorization? What if that information pertains to a public health concern, such as avian bird flu?

4. How difficult for your discipline is HIPAA to implement? How burdensome is it in terms of time and monetary cost?

5. Develop a discipline-specific patient informed consent checklist to use in clinical practice. If you are in a classroom setting, share the results.

REFERENCES, READINGS, AND RESOURCES

1. Bolles RN. *What Color Is Your Parachute?* Berkeley, CA: Ten Speed Press, 2006.

2. Cowan AE, Katz HS. HIPAA and the practice of law. *Texas Bar Journal.* 2004; December:962–963.

3. Health Insurance Portability and Accountability Act of 1996, 42 U.S.C. 1320.

4. Klitzman R. The quest for privacy can make us thieves. *New York Times.* May 9, 2006, A22.

5. Larsen EJ, Eaton TA. The limits of advance directives: A history and assessment of the Patient Self-Determination Act. *Wake Forest Law Review.* 1997;32:249–293.

6. Levy S. Searching for searches. *Newsweek.* Jan. 30, 2006, 34.

7. Patient privacy at risk in hospital hall ways, lobbies, cafeterias. *NEWS-Line for Occupational Therapists & COTAS.* 2004; October:12.

8. Rozovsky FA. *Consent to Treatment,* 2nd ed. Gaithersburg, MD: Aspen Publishers, Inc., 1990.

9. Scott RW. *Legal Aspects of Documenting Patient Care for Rehabilitation Professionals,* 3rd ed. Sudbury, MA: Jones and Bartlett, 2006.

10. Scott RW. *Professional Ethics: A Guide for Rehabilitation Professionals.* St. Louis: Mosby Year-books, Inc., 1998.

11. Scott RW. Guaranteeing patient rights: It's the law. *Advance for Directors in Rehabilitation.* 1992;Sept./Oct.:43–44.

12. Scott RW. Informed consent. *Clinical Management.* May/June 1991, 12–14.

13. Solomon J, King P. Waging war in the workplace. *Newsweek.* July 19, 1993, 30–34.

14. Wasserman R. Still hip to HIPAA? *Advance for PTs and PTAs.* 2004; November: 29–30.

15. Wollenhaupt G. Health care offers many entry-level opportunities. *Indianapolis Star.* Apr. 30, 2006, F7.

16. www.Kidzonline.org (streaming career self-assessment)

17. www.myersbriggs.org (fee-based guided personality self-assessment)

18. www.oln.org (Ohio Learning Network's values survey)

19. www.TipsforSuccess.org (professionalism survey)

Chapter 5

Seeking, Gaining, Retaining, and Thriving in Health Professional Employment

ABSTRACT

After a prospective health care professional has selected a target profession and completed entry-level educational requirements and any licensing or certification mandates, it is time to seek initial professional employment. The process of recruitment is a mutual process in which employers seek out and prospective employees respond to solicitations for employment. From the employee's perspective, the quality of the resume and the job interview are crucial for a successful outcome. In areas of critical employee shortage, such as medicine, nursing, and physical therapy, monetary incentives to work, including interviewing, relocation assistance, and sign-on bonuses, may be awarded. After being on the job, an employee must accomplish a wide range of complex, variegated tasks simultaneously, including, among others, acclimating to coworkers, superiors, meetings, and the organization's culture; overcoming the "learning curve;" assessing leadership styles and honing one's own leadership skills; taking an active role in performance appraisal (self and others); engaging in interpersonal negotiations on an ongoing basis; being productive; developing professionally and personally; and trying to be happy. Documentation of patient care is an important professional function for health care providers. It is as critically important as the rendition of care itself. The most important reason to document patient care activities is to record pertinent clinical information about the patient and to communicate it to other health care providers having an immediate need to know.

KEY WORDS AND PHRASES

- Absenteeism
- Acronym
- Appraisal
- Behaviorally anchored rating scales
- Benefits
- Breathing exercises
- Career ladder
- Compensation
- Constructive approach to discipline
- Cover letter
- Drucker, Peter
- Employee assistance program
- Employee discipline
- Employment agency
- Equal Pay Act of 1963
- Gender discrimination
- Graphic rating scales
- Incentives
- Informational interview
- Initialism
- Interpersonal bargaining
- Interview
- Management by Objectives

- Negotiation
- Networking
- Organizational culture
- Paid time off
- Pareto principle
- Patient care documentation
- Performance appraisal
- Portfolio
- Punitive approach to discipline
- Referral orders
- Rehabilitative approach to discipline
- Relaxation
- Relocation assistance
- Resume
- Retention officer
- Sandwich technique
- Satisficing
- Self-appraisal
- Spoliation
- Stress reduction
- Telephonic interview
- Theory of Career Anchors
- Total skills set
- Win–win outcome

OBJECTIVES

1. Prepare for initial or follow-on professional employment through meticulous self-assessment and organization, thorough research, and professional demeanor and comportment in the recruitment process.
2. Develop and maintain current an eye-catching and legally acceptable personal resume.
3. Practice effective self-monitoring and time management on the job.
4. Work well with others at all levels.

5. Negotiate effectively with others, bargain ethically and in good faith, and attempt to optimize negotiation outcomes for all involved persons and entities (i.e., seek "win–win" outcomes).

6. Be happy with yourself and your work but flexible enough to be able and ready to change jobs or careers whenever necessary.

You have finally completed your professional education, clinical affiliations, and licensing or certification requirements. The summit of health professional educational preparation has been reached. Now it is time to seek initial professional employment.

The process of seeking health professional employment begins with self-assessment. Important questions and review and research activities include the following:

1. Do I have a named prospective employer in mind? If so, how did you select the employer?

    a. Do I have more than one prospective employer in mind?

    b. What research have I conducted into prospective employers' businesses and opportunities?

    c. Have I networked with relevant people–resources yet?

    d. Do I have a resume ready for dissemination to prospective employers and others?

    e. Have I prepared cover, thank you, and follow-up letters for dissemination to prospective employers?

    f. Have I taken steps to ensure that my dress, comportment, and demeanor constitute the most professional presentation possible?

2. Where do you want to live as a health professional employee (country, region, town or city, neighborhood)?

    a. What is the relative cost of living in my selected site(s)?

    b. Do family, financial, or other obligations limit my geographic search area?

    c. Can I personally bear relocation costs without employer monetary relocation assistance?

3. What is my total skills set?

    a. Do my prior employment and volunteer experiences make me more marketable?

    b. What vocational skills, unrelated directly to my occupation, do I have?

    c. What languages, other than English (including American Sign Language), do I have at least elemental competence in?

4. What will it take to make me happy in my work?

5. Where do I hope and plan to be career-wise in 1, 3, 5, 10, and 25 years?

A prospective employee should carry out meticulous research into job markets and employers before soliciting employment. There are many ways to execute a successful job search, and all should be used when they are available. Colleges and universities where prospective employees are alumni offer placement services—some better than others; some are cost-free. Governments at all levels and private entities offer local job fairs throughout the year. The Internet offers an excellent and limitless database for job searches within a local area and far beyond, through information databases and online job banks. Networking with friends and business associates is often a very effective way to secure employment. Playing "foot detective," canvassing one's locale and soliciting informational interviews, is another means to the end. Employment agencies can help secure professional employment. Typically, these "headhunters" charge prospective employers, not job candidates, for successful placements.

Be sure to practice effective time and information management. There are a myriad of job search resources out there. Sometimes word-of-mouth recommendations from friends and colleagues who have used select services are the best tools to narrow the search.

Chapter Exercise 1

Create a top-10 list of what you think your best job search resources are. Be sure to vary the mix: colleagues, employment search agencies, Internet, in-person, and other resources.

Creating Your Resume

There seem to be an unlimited number of resume guides in the professional literature so as to make the task of resume preparation a daunting one. There are, however, common attributes to all successful resumes. Information is typically presented in reverse chronological order, from current to more remote data. A resume should present employment information in a functional format using active verb forms; that is, it should not only describe key job roles and tasks, but also the candidate's major accomplishments. For example, for a candidate with previous experience on a health care team, instead of just self-labeling the candidate as an "experienced team player throughout JCAHO (Joint Commission on Accreditation of Healthcare Organizations) survey process," cite instead what was specifically accomplished by the candidate, such as "singularly responsible for JCAHO departmental commendation during August 2005 survey." Be sure that the accomplishments cited are truthful and can be substantiated by others. Skills and accomplishments that are key to a given job position may be highlighted for eye direction and emphasis.

Similarly, educational accomplishments should be concisely written in a positive way so as to make the candidate maximally competitive. For example, if a candidate graduated *summa cum laude,* state and highlight that fact. Also, a candidate may selectively include quantitative data about grade point averages, when they are stellar (e.g., 3.5 out of 4.0 or above).

Specific references may be included at the bottom of a resume. Be sure to obtain prior approval from potential references before disseminating resumes. To do so is just common courtesy. Some sources will refuse to give a recommendation if they have not been contacted in advance. At least as often as listing references in a resume, the words "available upon request" are used. Prospective employers already know that candidates will provide references upon request, and thus, this commonly used phrase may seem a bit unnecessary.

Resumes posted on Internet sites must be digitally friendly. The electronic resume should fit the format of any site where it is posted, such as Jobs.Com or Monster.com. Discipline-specific key words are especially important for digital resumes. Be ready to include a tight, catchy qualifications summary (usually at the top of the resume) when called for. For site-specific guidance and for comparison, look at exemplars posted on that site.

Resumes present ethical, legal, and practical issues. From an ethical perspective, a resume must contain truthful information. If one "fudges" credentials or job details, then that dishonesty when discovered later is grounds for disciplinary action—even dismissal from employment. Legally, a resume cannot contain prohibited or precautionary information, such as age, disabilities, ethnicity, marital status, national origin, number of family members, race, religious affiliations, or sexual preference. The inclusion of such information is illegal

Summary of Resume Pointers

- Functional format
- Laser printed
- No legally prohibited or precautionary information
- Positive self-descriptive words and phrases
- Reverse chronological order
- Specific educational and vocational accomplishments
- Truthful information
- One to two pages
- 40-pound white bond paper

because it may form the basis for impermissible employment discrimination. Its inclusion on a resume in the United States may mean that the resume is discarded instead of reviewed for employment consideration. (This is not the case throughout much of the rest of the world, where such personal information is often standard resume information.)

From a practical standpoint, one should keep the length of a resume to one to two pages. Try to maximize "white space" on the paper so that your information is not too crowded. Human resource specialists screening resumes typically have less than 5 minutes per resume for their initial review, and thus, they are less inclined to expend substantial time on a more lengthy resume. Include quantitative data when appropriate.

A resume should be neatly laser printed on 40-pound white bond paper. Solicit review and frank critique of your resume from counselors and friends before disseminating it. Remember to use specifics when describing your accomplishments. Avoid self-descriptive words such as aggressive, competent, motivated, and reliable. These buzz words may create incorrect negative or less-than-optimal inferences about you. (Who wants someone for a job position who is *merely* competent?)

Chapter Exercise 2

In 30 minutes, draft a one-page resume seeking a hypothetical position as a physical therapist clinical manager with ABC Medical Center. Copy the resume onto an overhead slide to share with colleagues.

After a job candidate fields resumes to prospective employers, the next step in the recruitment process is to interview with prospective employers. Interview expenses are sometimes reimbursed by employers, especially when a candidate must undergo substantial expense to travel a long distance to interview on-site.

In some cases, telephonic job interviews or preinterviews are used by prospective employers. A telephonic interview is no less formal or nerve wracking than an in-person interview. It often leads to a crucial in-person job interview. When preparing for and carrying out a telephonic job interview, be sure to minimize distracters, such as a child crying or a dog barking, the flushing of a toilet, and rattling dishes. Under no circumstances should you use a cell phone because of potential signal disruptions. Be sure to sharpen your oral skills beforehand by practicing telephonic interviews with family or friends. In a telephonic interview, there is no opportunity for eye contact or visualizing body language, as in an in-person interview. Just as with an in-person job interview, be sure to follow-up by sending a thank you note, emphasizing your strengths for a given job position.

It is not always easy to obtain an interview. Often, you will have to make multiple attempts to reach a decision maker, such as a clinic department head. Be patient and persistent. Once identified, try to contact the person with whom an interview is desired at the most opportune times—perhaps at the beginning or end of a shift. Try not to connect with the prospective interviewer during the busiest times of the day.

After it is set, be sure to arrive 15 minutes early, and dress appropriately for your interview. Meena Thiruvengadam points out that dressing sexily in revealing clothes engenders a negative rather than positive impression of a candidate. Items of clothing such as too-tight pants or jeans for men and see-through blouses, micro-skirts, and ultra–high-heeled shoes for women are a no-no. Professionals are hired and retained for their expertise, not just to be "eye candy." Tasteful (although not necessarily ultraconservative) business attire for women and men that is clean and neatly pressed is always the safest bet!

> Dress appropriately. Professionals are hired and retained for their expertise, not just to be "eye candy."

During a job interview, whether before a group or single individual, remember to let the interviewer(s) set the agenda and pace for the session. Listen for important questions and be attuned to cues from the interviewer(s) and respond appropriately. Come ready to impart relevant research-based knowledge about the organization to showcase yourself as the best candidate for the position you seek—one who is well-prepared and poised and conveys important facts and details, when appropriate, about the organization during the interview.

Be prepared to respond during the interview to tough questions. Anticipate and practice (but do not memorize) your responses to these questions in advance. "Why did you not complete your college education?" "Explain the gaps in your employment history." "What are your weaknesses, if any?" "Describe your worst supervisor ever." "What do you bring specifically to this organization that makes you the perfect candidate?"

When cued by the interviewer, discuss compensation issues during the interview. If relocation assistance is sought, bring it up then and have a specific target amount in mind that can be justified with supporting data.

Follow the interview on the same or next day with a thank you note or letter. In that note or letter, re-convey your positive impressions of the organization, and restate your desire to hear from the interviewer regarding the position sought at his or her earliest convenience. Continue to follow up appropriately, without being labeled a pest.

Once hired, start off on the same good footing as during the interview. Dress appropriately for the job and arrive early. Be as attentive to the organization's needs as to your own. Be friendly and respectful to coworkers at all levels. To the extent possible, develop a sense of extended family within your work group and organization. This is the highly successful theory Z Japanese-style organization.

Every business organization has and evolves an organizational culture. Organizational culture consists of common beliefs and values that are manifested in a variety of ways, from work practices and organizational ethics to mottos and slogans to social functions and community outreach activities.

Always remember to practice basic etiquette and good manners in the office environment. Give and demand in return respect from colleagues. Accept responsibility for failures when justly deserved. As Farmer noted, character traits such as integrity, loyalty, and work effort cannot be taught. They can, however, be reflected upon and honed by every professional within an organization.

Vilfredo Pareto, an Italian economist (1848–1923), developed the 80/20 principle, which states that the first 20% of effort in furtherance of a task yields 80% of the total benefit derived from that task. By analogy, substantial monetary and nonmonetary resources are expended in recruiting and training employees. Their net value to any organization is not realized until the learning and cost curves associated with their in-house development are traversed, some 12 to 18 months after hire. To help keep these valuable human resources in place, many organizations have retention officers within human resource management departments to help, and many health care organizations employ career ladders to clarify and simplify professional employees' progression within the organization or system.

Consider the following example describing organizational culture:

Bayne-Jones Army Hospital on Fort Polk, Louisiana has, as part of its organizational culture, a quarterly staff recognition ceremony honoring civilian and military staff members who have excelled during that period of time. Virtually all staff—except those caring for patients at the time—are required to attend. The hospital commander calls awardees by name and position to the center of the cafeteria. Housekeeping staff stands shoulder to shoulder with medical service chiefs and receive their awards and the accolades of colleagues. Everyone understands each other's work and feels a little closer to one another by the end of the experience.

Management faces substantial challenges to keep key health care professionals in place and productive. According to a 2003 Commerce Clearing House survey of 436 human resource executives, as many as 11% of all employees are unhappy. For many, all goals seemingly have been accomplished. Stress is the purported cause for 45% of employees to quit their jobs. Vacation deprivation accounts for some $21 billion in unused vacation hours annually. Management challenges also include a mix of workers within which some 20% of the workforce are temporary workers, part-time and leased employees, and independent contractors, over whom managers necessarily exercise less control.

What keeps a valued professional employee within the organization? Schein's Theory of Career Anchors delineates self-perceived career goals for professionals. Among them are a desire to achieve and maintain professional competence, job security, and professional autonomy—the freedom to be creative and inventive in the work environment. Krueger theorized that worker satisfaction is a social phenomenon, primarily dependent on a subjective sense of meaning in one's work efforts. Lohr noted that counterbalancing employees' goals is the fact that employers want and demand productive, engaged workers. The trend is to award monetary incentives at the individual level based on performance, not seniority.

An area of potential concern for managers is team management. According to Brounstein, there are at least three areas of concern for team managers: responsibility, accountability, and conflict management. The stages of teamwork include forming (coming together and delineating roles), norming (setting down rules), storming (conflict), performing, and concluding.

A key requirement for success is to delineate a team's mission or purpose. Another is to have a concrete agenda. Team roles include, among others, a leader, whose duties include grabbing attendees' attention *ab initio* and forcing healthy debate on important issues under study, as well as a recorder, who takes notes and memorializes what is said and done.

There are several types of teams. Some are standing; some are *ad hoc*. Some teams are self-directed; that is, they have no supervisory oversight. Long-term teams, such as a rehabilitation department expansion committee, might have a schedule that includes daily check-in, weekly tactical meetings, monthly strategic meetings to analyze critical issues facing the team, and a quarterly off-site review, according to Lencioni.

Whether as part of a team or solo, you may have to present material to colleagues at a conference or meeting. Lubin and Mausy describe videoconferencing and virtual distance conferencing and their potential pitfalls. Cameras seem to magnify and exaggerate presenters' mistakes. Dress carefully if presenting remotely, as if before a live audience. Speak in a crisp conversational tone, and maintain eye contact with live and video conferees. Avoid culturally sensitive gestures, such as large hand and body movements, which tend to irritate listeners, especially Asians. Practice your presentation ahead of time to minimize nervousness. If your speaking voice is exceptionally soft, learn to speak more boldly.

Everyone at every level in an organization has the opportunity to step up to the plate as a leader, or change-agent for good, for the organization at some time in a career. In *The Seven Transformations of Leadership*, Rooke and Torbert shared the results of a 25-year survey of large corporations and governmental entities, including Deutsche Bank, Harvard Pilgrim Health Care, Hewlett-Packard, the National Security Agency, Volvo, and others. Respondents in the survey were asked to fill in word descriptors for the following sentence: "A good leader _____."

Rooke and Torbert delineated seven classes of organizational leaders, from least to most productive and complex. They pointed out that anyone can evolve along this leadership continuum with appropriate self-assessment and effective performance appraisal and mentoring.

At the bottom of the continuum are opportunists, leaders who strive to win any way possible. The opportunist is self-centered, but perhaps useful during crises. Five percent of leaders are opportunists.

Diplomats seek to avoid conflict by seemingly taking every side of an organizational issue. Although perhaps effective in a supporting role to unite factions, a diplomat is relatively ineffective as a leader. Twelve percent of organizational leaders are diplomats.

Experts (where most of us—especially in health care—reside) control information and knowledge. Experts make strong individualized contributions to organizational goals. Thirty-eight percent of leaders are expert–leaders.

Achievers represent classic managers that one might envision in any organization. They are goal oriented. They appropriately delegate authority to committees, teams, and work groups. Thirty percent of us are achievers.

Individualists "do it their way." They use unique approaches and methods to optimize employee performance and maximize productivity. The individualist may be a better fit in a large organization as a consultant than a general manager. Ten percent of leaders are individualists.

> Everyone at every level in an organization has the opportunity to step up to the plate as a leader or change agent for good for the organization at some time in a career.

Strategists are the personification of organizational change agents. They not only "get things done," but also generate individual, group, and organizational transformations while they promote mutual respect and gain throughout the organization. Four percent of leaders are strategists.

At the top of the ladder (where only 1% of leaders reside) are alchemists. The alchemist integrates company and societal goals and fosters social transformations. The alchemist is the personification of the true "Renaissance person."

Fandray points out that an effective leader must know the organization from top to bottom. The organizational leader must be willing to get his or her hands dirty, while not interfering unduly with subordinates' rhythm and flow. A good leader must also be able to facilitate and accept open, honest dialogue from employees. When the leader assents after an employee asks, "May I speak freely?" he or she must be prepared to hear and accept what the leader has given permission for subordinates to say.

Chapter Exercise 3

Assess your own leadership style according to Rooke and Torbert's continuum. Assess that of your current organizational leader and department head. Where do you go from here?

Performance appraisal is the process of periodically formally evaluating subordinates' performance, conducted by superiors. Performance appraisals by organizations are not required by law. Their purposes include accountability, rewarding positive performance, and identifying and correcting deficiencies in knowledge, skills, and abilities (KSAs). There are several popular types of performance appraisal instruments: self-appraisal through portfolios; forced-choice rating indicators, which include simple standards like "meets" and "doesn't meet" objectives; graphic rating scales (similar to visual analog pain scales); behaviorally anchored rating scales—richly annotated visual analog scales; and trendy but problematic 360-degree rating instruments, which include inputs from supervisors, peers, subordinates, patients, and perhaps others.

Key issues in performance appraisal systems include rater apathy and bias. In the central tendency effect, a rater tends to rate all employees within a narrow range around the average. The halo effect represents the situations in which raters label all ratees as either stellar or mediocre. A way to compensate for rater apathy or bias is for the organization to compile a rater profile, which clearly show how raters assess ratees over time. If too many fall within an extreme or at the center of the pack, then the credibility of the rater is suspect.

Chapter Exercise 4

Design a performance appraisal instrument for a hypothetical clinical manager (discipline unspecified) for a women's health clinic.

Management by objectives (MBO) was developed by Peter Drucker (1909–2005), a world-renowned business management theorist, in 1954. The most well-known management philosophy and appraisal system, MBO is a system in which there is joint responsibility between a rater and ratee for performance appraisal. Under MBO, a ratee and rater jointly establish major and minor performance objectives for the ratee; meet periodically (and *ad hoc*, as needed) during an appraisal period (typically 1 year) to assess progress and make changes, as necessary; and review results in a summative end-of-period appraisal interview. During the end-of-period appraisal interview, a rater carefully employs the "sandwich" assessment technique, constructively layering any negative comments between positive ones so as not to unduly injure the ratee's self-esteem. MBO is the antithesis of micromanagement.

Many managers procrastinate or avoid the performance appraisal process, in part because of its complexity. In a large organization, human resources management departmental consultants are available for help. Grensing-Pophal suggests that top-level managers consider linking management's compensation to the quality of performance appraisals of subordinates.

Employee compensation is an important motivator to morale, productivity, and especially retention of health care professionals. The three components of total compensation include salary (for overtime-exempt employees) or wages, benefits, and incentives. The Equal Pay Act of 1963 mandates that men and women be paid the same compensation for the same work. Nevertheless, study after study show that, particularly in health care, women doing the same work as men earn less compensation for their efforts. *Working Woman* magazine publishes an annual comparative salary survey, which consistently reveals substantial disparities in compensation between women and men doing the same work, particularly in health care service delivery. Consider monitoring this survey annually for data on your selected health care discipline.

Employee benefits were miniscule in the United States before the end of World War II (1945). They were referred to as "fringe" benefits because they typically only comprised 1% to 2% of the total compensation. Today, benefits make up 25% to 40% (or more, especially for high-level executives) of compensation. Mandatory benefits include three types of insurance coverage mandated by the federal and state governments: social security, unemployment compensation, and in most states (the others must self-insure for work-related injury payouts) worker's compensation. All other benefits—including vacation pay and health insurance for workers and their families—are permissive.

As a new health care professional, you should carefully consider negotiating with your employer (to the extent permitted by law and customary practice) over compensation and conditions of employment. There is very little individual bargaining in the United States over these items in the health care field (except for physicians). In the public sector (governmental employment), compensation and many key conditions of employment are firmly fixed by statutory law. In the private sector, however, they are normally subject to negotiation within a reasonable range. Unions do so all of the time, on behalf of groups of employees, or bargaining units. Employers fully expect professional employees to bargain over compensation and conditions of employment, and they do—in all endeavors except for health care. It is not unprofessional to negotiate with employers to improve one's compensation and working conditions.

Employee discipline is an important concern for workers and management. There are two foci of workplace disciplinary action—rehabilitative and punitive. These two foci are dependent on management philosophy. Rehabilitative discipline has the goal of remediating errant employees and returning them to full productive service. Punitive discipline strives to punish employees for infractions. Under either approach, a continuum of progressive discipline should optimally be used that fits the sanction to the offense. As the adage goes, "Let the punishment fit the crime."

A frequent reason for employee discipline is absenteeism. Vanderwall reported that the number one cause for employee absenteeism is family issues. Possible solutions for this problem, which costs employers nearly $1,000 per year per employee on average, include reconfiguration of vacation and holidays into global "paid time off" and onsite or otherwise readily available child and older person care for workers.

Another area of disciplinary concern is time abuse. Berglas delineates four types of chronic time abusers: people pleasers (social butterflies), perfectionists (those who seemingly never complete a task), pre-emptive time abusers (those with an entitlement mentality), and procrastinators (those who put work off over and over again until it is nearly too late). Most time abusers believe they are doing stellar work and deserve the down time they take as a reward.

Continuum of employee discipline (from least to most severe sanction):

1. Oral warning (advisement)
2. Written warning
3. Oral reprimand (chastisement)
4. Written reprimand
5. Suspension of perks (e.g., funded attendance continuing education experiences)
6. Suspension from work with pay
7. Suspension from work without pay
8. Review of and adverse action to clinical privileges
9. Punitive transfer (to a less desirable job or situs)
10. Punitive demotion (with resultant loss of pay)
11. Discharge from employment
12. Turning over evidence of possible criminal activity to licensing and certification boards and to the police

Jeffrey reported on employer monitoring of employee activities on the job. Seventy-six percent of employers open employees' mail received at work. It is an illegal and unethical invasion of privacy, however, to open any mail that is addressed to an employee and that is marked "personal." Fifty-five percent of employers monitor employees' activities on the Internet on company computers. Fifty-one percent monitor time on the phone to screen out personal calls. Thirty percent watch employees' time at computer keyboards, and 15% access employees' voice mail.

Employee assistance programs are available to employees with problems such as drug or alcohol abuse, family problems, and financial and psychological issues. Their purpose is to help employers keep valuable employees on the job and maintain high employee productivity. Employee participation in an employee assistance program is confidential, as is the reason for referral. Many businesses, including health care organizations and systems, are addressing employee and organizational problems and issues through workplace psychologists.

What can be done to assess why a good employee elects to leave the organization? Barada suggests using an exit interview. Some are conducted in-house, whereas others are done through an external agency (preferred). Exit interviews should be conducted 7 to 10 days after discharge, not on last day of the employee's work. Such interviews should be semistructured and include questions about what might have prevented valued employees from leaving. In all cases, interviewers should convey sincerity and express empathy over employees' situations and future.

Chapter Exercise 5

What if you have to terminate an employee with substantial longevity without cause, for example, because of downsizing staff in an outpatient clinic? How would you go about it?

Focus on Workplace Stress

Health care professionals perhaps face the greatest ongoing workplace stress of any professionals. Patients are of necessity in pain, demanding relief, and sometimes even dying before your eyes. It is not good to just admit and concede that high work stress is part of every health care professional's job.

Organizational pressure to achieve ever-increasing productivity, documentation and reimbursement demands, long work shifts, understaffing, and the practice constraints of managed care also contributes to health professional work-related stress. Forced to "do more with less," health care professionals at all levels run the risk of burning out from an overwhelming work environment. Personal life stressors make the situation even worse.

As a direct result, the quality of patient care delivery can suffer, while the likelihood of being sued can rise. Family and personal lives suffer as well.

Up to 40% of physicians feel burned out by the demands of the health care system, according to Romanski. Most health care professionals believe that administrative decision makers who demand 24/7/365 maximum productivity have little concept of what it really takes to care for patients and deal with the needs of their families and significant others. Manion asserts that health care professional burnout is the result of an accumulation of and overload from workplace and personal stressors.

Here are a few tips to help you manage stress and prevent burnout. Consider posting a list at work and passing it on to colleagues.

Know the Signs

Recognizing the warning signs of stress is the first step to learning how to manage it. Do not deny the existence and pressure of workplace and personal stress. Do not dismiss fatigue or forgetfulness as signs that you need more sleep or are just "getting old." These symptoms, along with detachment, difficulty making decisions, diminished productivity and sense of accomplishment, easy distractibility, and physical signs and symptoms such as headaches and back, joint, muscle, and neck pain, are all attributable to stress. If you find yourself on the verge of burnout, you may even begin to dread going to work each day. Do not start to work harder and longer to feel better. Instead, step back, assess your life and situation, and resolve to reduce your stress.

Adopt On-the-Job Strategies

Start with small things. Do "sweat the small stuff" in a positive way. For instance, make a point of greeting your co-workers with a smile and a friendly "hello" each day. This can help you feel better about being at work and pave the way for new and renewed friendships. Support your coworkers, too. If someone cannot get away for lunch, for instance, bring something back for him or her from the cafeteria or local deli. Not only is this a nice thing to do, but also your colleague may just return the favor at a later date when you most need some support.

Take on bigger issues as well. Ask your supervisor for help in resolving problems you may be having. You might, for instance, discuss how cumbersome patient care documentation has become or the fact that work hours are getting longer and yet you get the same number of breaks or none at all. During your discussion, you might suggest that your department meet on a regular basis—if it does not already—to work out other staff issues. Mention that weekly or monthly meetings might be helpful.

Try to take a physical break from work to clear your head. You might, for instance, take a walk around the parking lot for a few minutes each day.

Do not overlook the importance of going offsite altogether to attend continuing education courses. Not only will you receive valuable training, but you will also get a break from your regular routine.

Learn to Relax

Try some of the relaxation techniques that you may encourage your patients to use. For example, take time at home to listen to soft music or to meditate. Check out a good book or audiotape that teaches relaxation techniques, which include deep breathing and visualization. After you have experienced the relaxed state—in which your heart rate slows, your blood pressure drops slightly, and your muscles relax—you may be able to summon that feeling when it is needed at work.

Even if you do not master the more complex techniques of relaxation, some simple steps can be taken at work. If you are stressed out by an uncooperative patient or by an aide who is tuning you out, try taking a deep breath and counting to 10 instead of instantly reacting negatively. If it will take more than that to calm you down, return to your desk or another quiet place and take a few minutes to breathe in and out slowly while visualizing the release of stress from every part of your body.

Focus on Yourself

Part of reducing your stress hinges on taking good care of yourself. Eat healthy. Exercise regularly, and get enough sleep. Pamper yourself with a massage or a trip to a spa.

Evaluate whether your work level is worth the cost in stress and adjust accordingly. Money is not everything. Take up a hobby. Take your vacation and paid time off, and travel. You only live once. Have a support network of trusted colleagues, friends, and neighbors to turn to for advice and for "venting." Use or develop a sense of humor about your life and all that is in it.

By focusing on yourself and following the other tips outlined previously here you can keep your stress in check. By doing that, you will be able to maintain the high level of care that your patients expect—and deserve.

Focus on Interpersonal Negotiations

Everyone in every work setting is required to negotiate with others (or just give in) on an ongoing basis. It is best to approach interpersonal negotiations from a systematic standpoint. This section incorporates ideas from Fisher, Ury, and Patton's *Getting to Yes* (Penguin Books, 1992), the pre-eminent negotiations approach based on the 1980s Harvard Negotiation Project. This book is must reading for everyone in health care and is an easy read for quick studies. Published only in paperback, it can be digested cover to cover in less than an hour. For those whose appetite is whetted by reading the book, the Harvard Program of Instruction for Lawyers offers a two-course summer series on negotiations in Cambridge, Massachusetts, taught, along with others, by Roger Fisher. Many professionals other than lawyers (especially health care professionals) take these fine courses.

Before you ever negotiate with others over anything, you must have in your mind's eye a clear vision of what your personal bargaining objectives are and what the range of acceptable outcomes includes. After you have established these parameters, you are ready to engage in good-faith bargaining with "the other side."

The following are some of the salient bargaining tips for working with others to address and solve problems. All sides and individuals in bargaining must separate the participants in the bargaining process and their personalities from the problems and issues at hand. You are working together to battle a problem or set of problems—not each other. Stay objective in your presentations and discussions. Do not allow yourself to break down or become overly emotional during bargaining. Treat everyone in the process with equal respect. Listen more than you talk (the "51–49 rule"). Try, whenever possible, to quantify your positions and justifications. Most importantly, always bargain in good faith, that is, with a seriousness of purpose and a sincere desire to seek opportunities for mutual gain between and among all sides. Strive for a "win–win" outcome.

This "win–win" philosophy has recently been challenged by some authorities. It is argued that telegraphing the fact that one is seeking a mutually satisficing solution to a problem being negotiated over may actually impede successful bargaining. According to Lax, it may just be strategically better to keep your intentions in that regard under your cap.

Good negotiators listen effectively, are capable of persuading others to their side, and are competent strategists and tacticians. They also strive to create mutual value in their agreements with others and to ensure ownership of and joint responsibility for agreements reached in negotiations.

As part of negotiation strategy, focus as much on process (including the hows and whys of postagreement implementation of an agreement) as on outcome (making the deal). Make only realistic commitments within an agreement. Ask the tough questions about postagreement implementation early on to prevent the agreement from falling apart later on. Use a joint fact-finding team to prevent surprises.

Remember that informal background negotiations are as important as formal negotiations in sessions. In formal and informal negotiations, try to foster a sense of mutuality of need, and build mutual trust. Attach a price to maintaining the status quo. Offer incentives to bargain, when necessary. Engage in what Kolb and Williams label "process moves"—those required to break deadlocks or silence, seed fresh new ideas and perspectives, reframe issues and procedures, and build consensus toward creative solutions. Practice the Golden Rule by encouraging candor, confidentiality, and image preservation (face-saving) for all parties to negotiations.

As complex as it seems, you have been negotiating all along—hopefully relatively successfully—without much foresight, introspection, or training. With a little more reflection on the process of negotiation and some focused practice, you will do even better.

Focus on Patient Care Documentation

As part of the legal duty owed to patients, every primary health care provider is required by legal and professional and business ethical standards to record clinically pertinent history, examination, evaluative, and intervention-related information about their patients and to maintain that information in the form of patient treatment records. Besides primary health care providers (i.e., those licensed independent practitioners who can legally interact with patients without the requirement of a prior examination and referral by another health care provider), other health care professionals interacting with patients in supportive or consultative roles have the same duty to record patient information (if they are privileged under law and by their organizations to document) and ensure that it is safeguarded.

It is a truism that patient care documentation must be patient focused. Providers must use people-first, active-voice language when describing patients, both orally and in writing. Mrs. Jones, for example, is "a 52-year-old woman presenting with right CVA," not "a hemi."

Who can legally document information in patient records is a matter of federal and state law, organizational or systems policy, and customary practice. For inpatient records, therapeutic orders are normally written by medical physicians and surgeons attending individual patients. In most cases, no one except a physician can record information in the "Physician's Orders" section of an inpatient record, except where so permitted by law and custom, such as when a dental surgeon writes relevant orders for care for a specific patient. In outpatient patient care settings, however, especially in clinical settings in which no physician may be present, intervention orders are routinely written by primary health care providers other than physicians, for example, by physical therapists in direct access, or practice-without-referral, jurisdictions.

Patient care records take many forms. Two primary classifications of patient care records include inpatient records and ambulatory, or outpatient, records.

(Some authorities consider emergency treatment records as a separate category of patient care records.) Although in the past original patient treatment records were required by law to be handwritten in all jurisdictions, modernly, both inpatient and ambulatory records may now be created originally and maintained, either in whole or in part, on a computer.

> Documentation of patient care is as important as the rendition of care itself.

It is difficult to enunciate a precise definition for a patient care record. In simplest terms, a patient care record is a memorialization of a specific patient's health status at a given point in time. The patient treatment record includes clinically pertinent information that is clear, concise, comprehensive, individualized, accurate, objective, and timely. It serves both as a business document and as the legal record of care rendered to the patient.

From business and clinical perspectives, as well as from a legal standpoint, documentation of patient care is as important as the rendition of care itself. This axiom holds true for the protection of patients and health care professionals alike. For health care providers, patient care documentation is substantive evidence of the nature, extent, and quality of care rendered to patients, whereas for patients, it serves as a permanent record of their health status, which may, among many other purposes, serve as a historical record for future life-saving intervention.

Purposes of Patient Care Documentation

The patient care record serves a myriad of important purposes. Primary health care professionals and health care organizations act as fiduciaries, or persons and entities in a special position of trust *vis a vis* patients under their care. Therefore, logically, the primary purpose of patient care documentation is to communicate vital information about a patient's health status to other health care providers concurrently caring for that patient and having an imminent need to know the information contained therein. This principle operates either in an inpatient or outpatient care setting. The clinical information entered by one health care professional in a patient's record is assimilated by other providers into their intervention plans and incorporated with their goals for patients to ease discomfort, speed recovery, and maximize function and independence.

Despite what may be suspected by some to be the primary purpose for patient care documentation—self-protection from patient-initiated claims and litigation—this is clearly not the case. That kind of negative approach to documentation serves no positive purpose and only instills fear in health care professionals. Such fear, in turn, fosters an atmosphere of costly defensive health care practice.

A defensive posture regarding patient care documentation may actually increase the chances of malpractice exposure. Patients and their significant others can readily sense a health care provider's defensiveness. They justifiably find distasteful the kind of formal, cold, business-like relationship that inherently results when a health care professional puts fear of malpractice exposure (or other self-interest, such as revenue maximization) ahead of the patient's welfare. If patients come to believe that their health care providers are excessively focused on self-protection from litigation exposure or other selfish considerations, then they may be more inclined to pursue legal actions if and when an adverse outcome results from intervention.

There are many other important purposes for patient care documentation. Documentation of patient care serves as a basis for planning and for ensuring continuity of care in the future for patients currently under care, particularly for those inpatients who, after discharge, will require health professional intervention at home. By memorializing a patient's health status at any given point, documentation also serves to create a historical record of a given patient's health, from which data can be extracted for and used in future contingencies, ranging from emergent life-threatening crises to disability determinations.

Documentation also forms the basis for monitoring and assessing the quality of care rendered to patients as part of a quality management program. Such programs are required of health care facilities accredited by entities such as the Joint Commission on the Accreditation of Healthcare Organizations (Joint Commission), the Commission on Accreditation of Rehabilitation Facilities (CARF), the National Committee on Quality Assurance (NCQA), and others, including local, state, and federal public oversight entities.

Besides its utility as a database for monitoring and evaluating the quality of patient care, patient care documentation is useful as a productivity measure of provider workloads and to assess whether health care providers are practicing effective utilization management of human and nonhuman health care resources. It also serves, through identifying deficiencies, to ascertain whether there are needs for training for health care providers, from communication skills to substantive aspects of patient care.

As a business document, the patient care record is also evaluated by governmental third-party payer entities such as Medicare, Medicaid, TriCare (for military beneficiaries), and state and local governmental entities and by insurance companies and other third-party payers to determine levels of reimbursement for patient care. Documentation of patient care, then, is the primary means of justifying reimbursement for treatment. The treatment record also provides information that is useful for scientific and clinical research and for education.

Besides being a business document, the patient care record is a legal document as well. In the event of a health care malpractice claim or lawsuit, providers' documentation of patient care activities provides substantive and relatively objective evidence of the care that was rendered to the patient claiming malpractice. Documented evidence of care recorded in the patient's record provides expert witnesses with a basis from which to form a professional opinion on whether a provider or multiple providers met or violated standards of practice and legal standards of care. Patient care documentation also serves many other legal functions, including, among others, its use as substantive evidence of work or functional capacity in worker's compensation and similar administrative proceedings.

As an additional legal issue, documentation of patient informed consent protects patients, providers, and health care organizations and systems by serving as written evidence that a patient actually understood the risks and benefits of specific interventions and made a knowing, informed choice to undergo examination and accept recommended interventions. Documentation of a patient's desires in the event of that patient's mental incapacitation through advance directives serves also to memorialize patient decisions, evidence respect for patient autonomy, and protect health care professionals who must carry out the patient's valid advance directives.

Purposes of Patient Care Documentation

1. Communicates vital information about a patient's health status to other health care providers concurrently caring for that patient and having an imminent need to know the information contained therein.

2. Acts as a basis for patient care planning and continuity of care.

3. Serves as the primary source of information for assessing the quality of patient care rendered.

4. Provides information for reimbursement and utilization review decisions.

5. Identifies provider deficiencies and training needs.

6. Serves as a resource for research and education.

7. Serves as a business document.

8. Serves as a multipurpose legal document.

9. Provides substantive evidence on whether providers' care rendered, and health care organizations' oversight of patient care activities, met or violated legal standards of care.

10. Memorializes patient informed consent to examination and intervention, as well as patient desires regarding life-sustaining measures in the event of a patient's subsequent mental incapacitation, through advance directives.

Contents of Patient Care Records

Required contents of patient care records vary greatly, depending on, among other considerations, state and federal laws and regulations, accreditation standards, organization and system requirements, and patient care settings. For hospitalized patients, for example, patient records are typically divided into two parts: (1) intake, or admissions, data, including the relevant patient histories and assessments, physical examinations by admitting physicians (including admission studies and tests) and other primary health care professionals, and the admission diagnosis or diagnoses, and (2) the clinical record, in which progress notes, consultations, laboratory tests, diagnostic imaging studies, operative and anesthesia reports, and discharge summaries are written. Contents of outpatient records display greater variation.

Formats for Patient Care Documentation

Because communication of patient information to other health care professionals concurrently caring for that patient is of such critical importance, clinicians must ensure that their documentation of a patient's health status is understood by others on the health care team. This section discusses acceptable formats for communicating patient information to others. Practical considerations for effective documentation are considered in the next section.

There are practically only three general patient care documentation formats: narrative format, template (or report) format, and acronym/initialism format. The simplest form of patient care documentation is in narrative, or free-form, format. The prose form of literary composition, used by students in papers, theses, and dissertations, is the most common example of narrative format. Template or report format uses word and phrase prompts and blank spaces to generate and record data. Most computerized documentation systems are primarily in template format. The acronym/initialism format employs alphabetic letters to form words (acronyms) or initialize data. "SOAP" is an example of the acronym format; "P-S-P" (Problem-Status-Plan) is an example of initialism format. The three basic patient care documentation formats may be combined into hybrid formats, and all three are equally amenable to accession to the computer medium.

"SOAP" was originally developed by Dr. Lawrence Weed at the University of Vermont in the late 1960s to standardize physician and nursing documentation. It is part of the highly structured problem-oriented medical record system.

Each of these three formats offers relative advantages and disadvantages. The principal advantages of the narrative format are that it is the most flexible of formats and does not limit the amount of data that writers can annotate. Its disadvantages are that it does not compartmentalize information into readily discernible categories and that it facilitates verbosity by writers. The template or report format's key advantages are that information is neatly compartmentalized and standardization is maximized through its use. Its disadvantages include that it may facilitate underdocumentation (e.g., when all blank spaces are not addressed) and that special circumstances may be difficult to address or may be relegated to a miscellaneous section on the form. Acronym/initialism formats share the compartmentalization advantage that characterizes the template or report format. SOAP format (discussed in greater detail later here) is so universally used by health care providers and organizations that its use may facilitate faster processing of information by users and thus enhance communication.

The problem-oriented SOAP approach highlights key information, including historical information about a patient and his or her chief complaint, clinical examination findings and objective observations of the examining clinician, the diagnosis (or diagnoses) or evaluative findings, and a proposed plan of intervention for the patient. In essence, both acronym/initialism and template/report formats are problem oriented. Narrative patient care documentation, on the other hand, often makes critical patient information difficult to locate expeditiously.

More on SOAP

In SOAP format, patient information is compartmentalized into four main sections of an initial note: the subjective element ("S"), the objective element ("O"), the assessment ("A"), and the plan ("P"). Collectively, these elements comprise the problem-oriented SOAP note documentation model. Under the SOAP note format, health care professionals can quickly access pertinent information recorded by another provider who conducted a prior examination of a patient by referring to the four elements of the SOAP note.

The "S," or subjective, element of a rehabilitation-setting initial SOAP note includes the following information: (1) a patient's medical diagnosis (or diagnoses); (2) a summary of the patient's relevant health history taken from the patient interview and from a review of the patient's available records; (3) the patient's expression of his or her condition, including parameters of symptoms, such as the location, quality (sharp, dull, throbbing), severity (minimal, moderate, severe along a visual analog scale), nature (constant, intermittent), and factors that increase or decrease pain; the presence or absence of sensory symptoms (e.g., paresthesia, anesthesia, and loss of normal proprioception [perception of joint position in space]); ambulation, balance, and coordination status; level of independence; and mental status; and (4) the patient's medication list, subjective reactions to medications being taken, and any allergies—documented or reported. Some clinicians create a separate section for the patient history and do not include it under the "S" element of a S-O-A-P note.

Many patients provide a medication list, which becomes part of the examination documentation. Providers usually write "See attached list," rather than taking the time to write out all patient medications. Providers are cautioned to monitor carefully patients/medication lists, especially for medications that providers know, or should know, have been withdrawn from the market.

The "O" element of the rehabilitation-setting initial S-O-A-P note includes objective examination data and findings about the patient. These data might include skin appearance and tone; muscle, sensory, and neurological examination results; the patient's activities of daily living status; results of a gait analysis; analytical skills test results; reflex test findings; and laboratory test and diagnostic imaging report results.

The "A" element of the rehabilitation-setting initial S-O-A-P note represents the evaluating health care professional's clinical assessment, based on objective examination findings and subjective input from the patient and others and on available patient health records.

The "P" element of the rehabilitation-setting initial S-O-A-P note delineates the clinician's intended plan of intervention for the patient. In this section, the clinician might also document that the patient gave informed consent to the examination and recommended intervention. If, in addition to being examined, the patient receives initial treatment or other intervention, then the objective and subjective results of such intervention should also be summarized under the "P" element of the initial note.

A fifth alphabetical initial may be added to the traditional S-O-A-P format, that being a "G" for functional goals. As outcome criteria, functional goals represent expectations of and for a patient regarding the patient's ability to carry out important activities of daily living. These goals are often subdivided into short-term goals (often abbreviated STG) and long-term goals (LTG).

Do Stated Treatment Goals Equate to a Legally Binding "Therapeutic Promise"?

A legal issue that sometimes arises in health care malpractice proceedings is whether patient goals established by a clinician in a patient care note represent a guarantee, or warranty, of a specific therapeutic result, for which the failure to achieve the goal may be labeled a breach of a therapeutic promise, resulting in contract-based liability on the part of the provider and/or health care organization. The answer to this question is generally no. Patient intervention goals are not promises made to a patient but, rather, are the written manifestation of the health care provider's professional judgment. As such, goals merely represent the provider's professional opinion about expected outcomes of intervention. Health care providers are cautioned, however, that the actual communication of specific therapeutic promises to patients may create a binding legal obligation to meet the promises made or to face liability for breach of contract if they are not achieved.

Summary of S-O-A-P-G Initial Patient Care Notation Format

S: Contains historical information (medical, medication, occupational, familial, and social) relevant to a specific patient's health condition or complaint, related by the patient to the primary health care professional and extracted from the patient's health record.

O: Contains the results of examination findings, including relevant laboratory and diagnostic imaging results.

A: Contains the evaluative assessment and clinical diagnosis/diagnoses.

P: Contains the proposed plan of intervention for the patient and may include documentation of the patient's informed consent to examination and intervention and receipt of HIPAA information. If initial intervention ensues, then a summary of results of initial care is also recorded.

G: Contains short- and long-term functional goals (patient-generated expected functional outcomes) of intervention.

Problem-Status-Plan Initialism Format

A variation of the SOAP problem-oriented patient care documentation format often used for recording patient progress notes is the Problem-Status-Plan, or "P-S-P" format. Under this format, a re-evaluation note will include the patient's problem(s) and prior evaluative findings and diagnosis (or diagnoses) under "P", the patient's subjective expression of his or her condition after treatment and the objective findings of the re-examination are listed under "S", and the revised plan of intervention is listed under the second "P." As with the SOAP format, some clinicians prefer to add a "G" element to this format as well, to memorialize their revised outcome criteria, or functional goals, based on the patient's activities of daily living/work-related needs and desires.

Problem-Status-Plan (P-S-P) Documentation Format for Patient Re-evaluations

P: Contains a summary of the patient's prior evaluative findings and diagnosis (or diagnoses).

S: Contains subjective and objective information about the patient's condition on re-examination.

P: Contains the modified patient intervention plan, based on the current clinical findings.

No one format is "the" correct format for meeting the required legal standard of care for patient care documentation. As long as a particular format used by health care professionals working in concert promotes effective communication about their patients' health and conditions, then the format is legally acceptable and within the legal standard of care. Considerations of third-party payer documentation requirements for reimbursement, although not a health care malpractice legal issue per se, are critically important, too, for the financial viability of health care professionals, organizations, and systems. Existing and developing computerized documentation formats facilitate the simultaneous compliance with regulatory (particularly HIPAA) and procedural documentation requirements of multiple third-party payers and are highly recommended for use by providers and facilities.

Risk Management Considerations for Effective Patient Care Documentation: The First Draft Is the Final Work Product

Imagine that you are an author of fiction novels. Several hours after signing a "contingent" book contract based on an outline proposal, your prospective publisher calls you on the telephone and demands that you begin writing immediately and submit a final product within 1 week. As an added burden, imagine that the publisher tells you that you will be allowed only one draft of the novel, on which a firm publication decision will be based. Impossible? Ludicrous?

Now imagine that you are a health care provider working in the emergency department of a regional trauma center. A critically injured patient is transported to your facility without notice. While other members of the team begin to examine the comatose patient, you begin to record the patient's vital signs on an admission form. The patient suddenly goes into cardiac arrest, and cardiopulmonary resuscitation immediately ensues. With all of the tension and haste inherent in this situation, your recording of the information shouted to you by surgeons and nurses reflects your state of nervousness. The entries are scribbled, and words, syllables, and rough diagrams take the place of full sentences and careful illustrations that otherwise would be standard procedure.

Now imagine that the patient's condition deteriorates, and she dies while in the emergency department. A health care malpractice lawsuit is filed, and it proceeds to trial. The attorney for the patient's estate and her survivors offers the emergency room admission record into evidence. The conduct of the medical team will probably be judged in large part on the basis of that record of care that, of necessity, was written in an atmosphere of haste and tension, without any opportunity for drafts or revisions. Similar circumstances occur in emergency departments, operating suites, and other locations throughout health care organizations literally tens of thousands of times each day.

Although not every patient care encounter demands that documentation of care be conducted "under the gun," in almost every situation health care clinical professionals interacting with patients are prohibited from revising or refining their initial examination or intervention patient care entries because to do so would constitute *spoliation*, or the intentional destruction or alteration of patient care documents with the specific intent to hide or change their clear meaning. The conduct of health care providers, unlike with most other professionals, is routinely evaluated and judged on the basis of a first "draft" of their work product—that is, the patient care record.

Patient Care Documentation Problems, Errors, and Suggestions

Because the consequences of patient care documentation entries are so critically important to effective management of health care malpractice risk exposure, this section presents 25 common patient care documentation problems, errors, and suggestions, designed to minimize the incidence and effects of incomplete or legally substandard documentation. Some of the problems identified herein may seem so trivial and their solutions so obvious that they do not merit mentioning; however, very often in health care malpractice proceedings, the simplest, seemingly trite documentation mistakes have the most serious adverse impact on legal case outcomes. No one should think that his or her intelligence is being insulted by some of these apparently simplistic guidelines for patient care documentation because the recommendations presented may help to prevent a finding of liability for health care malpractice and all its adverse consequences.

Twenty-Five Documentation Problems, Errors, and Suggestions

1. Documentation problem: illegible notation
2. Documentation error: failure to identify (or correctly identify) the patient under care
3. Documentation error: failure to annotate the date (and time, depending on customary practice) of patient care activities
4. Documentation problem: use of multiple or inconsistent documentation formats by providers in a facility

(continued)

5. Documentation error: failure to use an indelible instrument to record examination, evaluation, diagnostic, prognostic, intervention, or outcome data about a patient under care

6. Documentation problem: pen runs out of ink midway through a patient care record entry

7. Documentation problem: line spacing in patient care record entries

8. Documentation problem: signing patient care record entries

9. Documentation problem: error correction

10. Documentation error: unauthorized and unrecognized abbreviations

11. Documentation errors: use of improper spelling, grammar, and the use of extraneous verbiage not affecting patient care

12. Documentation problems: physician orders: transcription problems; examining and intervening on behalf of patients without written orders, where legally required

13. Documentation error: untimely documentation of patient care activities

14. Documentation error: identifying or filing an incident report in the patient care record

15. Documentation problem: failing to delineate patient care rendered or identify clinical information supplied by another provider

16. Documentation error: blaming or disparaging another provider in the patient care record

17. Documentation error: expressing personal feelings about a patient or patient family member or significant other in the patient care record

18. Documentation suggestion: document observations and findings objectively

19. Documentation suggestion: document with specificity

20. Documentation error: recording *hearsay* ("second-hand" input) as fact

21. Documentation suggestion: Exercise special caution when countersigning another provider's, student's, or intern's patient care notation

22. Documentation error: failure to document a patient's informed consent to examination and intervention

23. Documentation suggestion: document thoroughly patient/family/significant other understanding of, and safe compliance with, discharge, home care, and follow-up instructions

24. Documentation suggestion: carefully document a patient's noncompliance with provider directives or recommendations

25. Documentation suggestion: carefully document a patient's or family member/significant other's possible contributory negligence related to alleged patient injuries or lack of progress

Documentation Problem: Illegible Notation

If there is one comment that patients make most often, it probably is that their physicians and other health care providers do not write legibly in patient health records. It might not surprise you to hear that health care professionals themselves also often cannot decipher one another's patient care record entries, causing them either to have to consult with the writer of an entry for "translation" or, worse yet, to disregard the illegible information or even an entire entry.

Even in emergency situations, there is no excuse for documenting patient care illegibly. Keep in mind that the primary purpose of patient care documentation is to communicate vital information about a patient to other health care professionals concurrently caring for that patient and having an imminent need to know.

How many times have you had to struggle to try to decipher another health care provider's handwriting on an intervention order, in a consultation report, or in another document? Have you ever had to spend time trying to decipher your *own* prior patient care entries? Assuming that the latter situation has occurred on at least one occasion for all of us, imagine how embarrassing it would be to be asked by a patient's attorney during a deposition to read one of your own garbled notation entries and not be able to do so, or worse yet, to be asked to read it aloud before a judge, a jury, and 40 to 50 spectators at trial. The devastating effect that such a situation would have on a health care malpractice defendant—health care provider's or organization's case is self-evident.

Clinical managers and health care organization and system administrators must take whatever administrative steps are necessary to ensure that health care professionals within their domains of supervision and control write legibly. This may entail developing alternative documentation systems not based on handwritten notation for providers who cannot be made compliant. For example, the use of dictation and transcription of entries is a viable alternative to handwritten documentation for such primary health care professionals. The use of computerized documentation systems can also alleviate the problem of illegible patient care documentation. When these systems are unavailable, individual providers who cannot write or print legibly should type their patient care entries. As a last (and drastic) resort, the retention of clinical privileges in a facility can and should be conditioned on the ability to communicate legibly with other providers and support personnel.

> When a health care provider's illegible documentation of patient care information is the proximate cause of delayed treatment or patient injury, the failure to communicate effectively constitutes actionable health care malpractice.

Providers themselves should also self-police to ensure that their handwritten patient care documentation is legible and neat. When necessary, print or type entries instead of writing in cursive. Remember that a negligent failure to communicate patient treatment information is itself a form of health care malpractice and a legitimate basis for primary (direct) liability for resultant patient injury.

Documentation Error: Failure to Identify (or Correctly Identify) the Patient Under Care

Failure to identify, or correctly identify, a patient under care in documentation is another form of negligence that can lead to malpractice liability. Every page of a patient's record must contain the patient's full name written in indelible ink or in the form of a stamp. Each page should also contain appropriate personal identifying information about the patient to facilitate expedient communication with the patient or relevant others.

As a primary health care provider or supportive professional writing patient information on a document, you bear primary ethical and legal responsibility for ensuring that the patient written about is correctly identified on the document. As a matter of customary practice, do not relinquish control over a piece of paper involving patient care that you have written an entry on unless the patient's name and identifying information is on it.

Documentation Error: Failure to Annotate the Date (and Time, Depending on Customary Practice) of Patient Care Activities

Failure to annotate the date (and, where required, the time) of patient care can be a supporting factor in the imposition of health care malpractice liability. Accounting for the chronology of patient care is especially crucial for physicians and nurses administering medications to patients when a duplicate dose of the medication in issue might be toxic to the patient. Providers such as physical and occupational therapists, whose practice and utilization management standards set limits for the number of permissible interventions in a given time period, must also carefully annotate the dates (and perhaps times) of interventional activities. Date entries must always include the day, month, and year. To avoid confusion over a.m. and p.m. where treatment times are annotated, consider adopting the systematic use of military time (e.g., 0001 to 2400 hours).

Documentation Problem: Use of Multiple or Inconsistent Documentation Formats by Providers in a Facility

Effective communication of patient care information among health care providers is most efficaciously facilitated when providers all "sing from the same sheet of music." Clinical managers, department and service chiefs, and facility/system administrators must ensure that providers are using documentation formats that are universally understood by other providers in the facility/system where the relevant documentation may be used. The best way to ensure this is to standardize documentation formats, requiring primary health care providers, for example, to use the SOAP (Subjective-Objective-Assessment-Plan) format for initial patient examination notation and the P-S-P (Problem-Status-Plan) format for patient follow-up and discharge notation. Alternatively, a facility or system may mandate the use of a common template or series of template forms for patient care documentation. Obviously, some degree of flexibility must be built into any standardized documentation system; however, the use of enigmatic formats or data by individual providers should be prohibited as a matter of policy. If professional colleagues cannot decipher your patient care notation, "What we have here is a failure to communicate."

Documentation Error: Failure to Use an Indelible Instrument to Record Examination, Evaluation, Diagnostic, Prognostic, or Outcome Data About a Patient Under Care

Another commonplace documentation error involves the use by providers of writing instruments other than indelible ink, such as pencils, erasable ink, and felt-tipped pens, whose patient care entries are easily obliterated or smeared. When patient care entries are made in pencil or erasable ink, the temptation to "correct" or otherwise alter entries—especially in the face of a potential legal action—is heightened. As a preventive measure for the protection of all concerned, do not write or allow providers under your control to write patient care entries in any medium except indelible (black or dark blue) ink. Even where there is no evidence of alteration or spoliation of records in a health care malpractice case, an inference of negligence might be ascribed by a jury or judge to a facility in which the use of erasable notation is tolerated.

In a similar vein, always ensure that computerized patient care entries are saved on the computer before leaving the relevant software program. Administrators should systematically provide for "automatic save" features to prevent the loss or subsequent alteration of crucial patient care data when an operator leaves a computerized patient care documentation program.

Documentation Problem: Pen Runs Out of Ink Midway Through a Patient Care Entry

What do you do if, when writing a patient care entry, your pen runs out of ink? Well, obviously you must complete the entry with a second pen (hopefully with the same color ink). You should precede the second part of the entry, however, with a brief parenthetical phrase, stating that your first pen ran out of ink at that point. Be sure to initial the parenthetical comment. The parenthetical comment is necessary to prevent a later inference of spoliation of records in the event of any legal action involving the patient in whose record patient care activities are being documented. An example of how to document a change in writing instrument partway through documenting an entry appears in Exhibit 5–1.

Exhibit 5–1   Documenting a Necessary Change of Writing Instrument During a Patient Care Record Entry

Consider the case in which a registered nurse's pen runs out of ink midway through the entry of a narrative-format nursing progress note made at a shift change. The change in pens used to write would be documented as follows:

Nov. 23, 200x/1445: Patient resting comfortably. Dyspneic breathing/(Note: Original pen ran out of ink. M.K.M., R.N.)/no longer observed. Normal skin color.

RR = 14/min. (signature and title).

Documentation Problem: Line Spacing in Patient Care Record Entries

Spoliation, or intentional malicious alteration of patient health records, is a growing problem with serious ethical and legal implications for health care professionals and organizations. One effective method that clinical managers and facility/system administrators can use to decrease the temptation on the part of providers to add information to prior entries is to establish a policy requiring that providers documenting patient care write on every line.

Documentation Problem: Signing Patient Care Record Entries

By signing (or initialing) a patient care entry, a provider authenticates and acknowledges legal and professional ethical responsibility for the information contained in the entry. It goes without saying that one should have special pride in his or her signature, and thus, providers are urged to sign patient care entries legibly and neatly. From a risk management perspective, a legible and neat signature may also serve to create a positive impression in the minds of others reviewing the record. In the event of a subsequent health care malpractice proceeding involving the record, a judge and jury viewing a record with a neat signature may rightly conclude that its author was as careful and precise in caring for the patient–litigant as in signing his or her name.

Along with one's signature, the author of a patient care entry should include his or her professional title (e.g., COTA, CPO, DC, DO, LPN, MD, NP, OTR, PA, PT, PTA, RD, RN, SLP). Irrespective of how neat a signature is, a stamp with the provider's full legal name and title should be affixed in the vicinity of the signature. State or federal law, facility/system policy, and local or national customary practice may dictate inclusion of other information in a legal signature, including the provider's professional license number.

State or federal law also dictates whether a rubber stamp impression of a provider's signature or a computer-generated electronic signature constitutes a valid legal "signature."

Documentation Problem: Error Correction

To err is human. To correct errors properly in patient care records is good risk management. Despite a good-faith effort to document accurately the first time around, everyone will make mistakes occasionally when documenting patient care data. Mistakes can range from using an incorrect term in an entry to writing a patient's entry on a page labeled with another patient's personal data.

Individual health care professionals who write patient care entries, clinical managers, and facility/system administrators should develop standardized rules for correcting patient care entries in records and on other official documents. One method that is commonly used is to draw (or trace along a straight-edge) a single line neatly through the erroneous material and then initial it. Providers should also consider indicating the date and time of the correction, even though error correction normally is made during the same sitting as the original erroneous entry.

A basic rule that must be obeyed is to avoid hiding a mistake. Do not obliterate any patient care entry by scratching out what is written. Do not erase any entry. Similarly, the use of correction liquid to obliterate a prior entry in patient care records is a prohibited method of error correction. The purpose of patient care record error correction is to prevent a potential miscommunication of information, not to hide or obliterate what is being edited.

Even writing over an entry a second time for the innocent purpose of making lighter ink more readable is discouraged, because a patient–plaintiff's attorney or a judge or jury reviewing the record at a later date may reasonably be suspicious that an improper entry alteration had occurred. Ensure that what you write in a patient's record is clear, bright, and neat the first time.

Criminologists are expert at detecting alteration of patient care record entries, and such evidence, in the face of a denial of record alteration, is devastating to a health care professional's credibility generally and to the defense case in health care malpractice proceedings. Specialists can readily distinguish the ink from two different pens, even when the color appears identical to the naked eye, and can even opine on whether entries were made at different times on the basis of penmanship and writing style.

What should a provider involved in a health care malpractice case say if he or she has committed an error in patient data entry correction, such as obliterating a prior entry? By all means, the provider concerned must coordinate with legal counsel on what specifically to do and say about the mistake during deposition, at trial, or otherwise. In all cases, he or she must not deny the mistake if asked about it during official proceedings. To do so would be to give false testimony—a criminal offense in most cases.

Authorities writing on the subject recommend different approaches to commenting on why error correction is being carried out. One acceptable method of correcting patient care entry errors is simply to draw through the erroneous material and initial and date the deletion, as discussed previously here. Some authorities recommend the commonly used technique of handwriting the word *error* above the correction. Others urge providers not to use the word *error* to prevent an inference of clinical negligence associated with the entry error from arising in a judge or jury's mind. Some authorities recommend using words such as mistake or mistaken entry ("M.E.," if this is a recognized abbreviation), instead of "error." Still others recommend writing a brief note in the margin adjacent to the correction indicating why it was made. The most prudent approach to annotating error corrections is to avoid it altogether, so as not to create an adverse inference of sloppy patient care in the minds of judges or juries in health care malpractice proceedings.

> The purpose of patient care notation error correction is to prevent a potential miscommunication of information, not to hide or obliterate what is being edited.

Documentation Error: Unauthorized and Unrecognized Abbreviations

In the busy managed care environment of contemporary patient care, nothing is more at a premium than time. Using acceptable abbreviations in patient care notation is a smart way to facilitate communication and save precious minutes that writing each and every term and phrase out long-hand would entail. The selective use of abbreviations facilitates communication and improves patient care because it is easier for other providers caring for a patient being written about to scan shorter notes containing known abbreviations than to labor through longer narratives without abbreviations.

Clinicians, however, need to exercise caution when using abbreviations to ensure that others understand what information they intend to convey. To ensure uniformity and universal comprehension, clinical, facility, and system managers must develop standardized lists of approved abbreviations and require providers to use only those abbreviations. The list or lists of facility-approved abbreviations must be widely disseminated to all those personnel who do or might write, interpret, transcribe, and review patient care notation, including clinicians, students, medical records personnel, and administrative, secretarial, and clerical personnel.

Facility/system administrators should seek broad input from all potential users when formulating the lists and must ensure that approved abbreviations lists remain current. An ongoing systematic review of existing approved abbreviations is highly recommended.

Special caution must be exercised when one abbreviation may have two or more common meanings, such as "AC," for acromioclavicular, alternating current, or anterior cruciate. If the intended meaning for such an abbreviation is not clear to potential readers, then the writer must spell the word out to ensure comprehension by all.

The potential adverse consequences of using unintelligible abbreviations can be as serious as carrying out patient care in a negligent manner. If providers relying on cryptic patient care documentation misinterpret vital patient information and take injurious courses of action toward a patient as a result, then both the drafter and reader of that erroneous information may face health care malpractice liability.

Documentation Errors: Improper Spelling, Grammar, and the Use of Extraneous Verbiage Not Affecting Patient Care

As with illegible notation, improper word spelling and the use of incorrect grammar by health care professionals reflect negatively on them individually and on departments, services, facilities, and systems. These vocabulary errors may create an impression of carelessness, which, if inferred and extrapolated by judges or juries in health care malpractice legal cases, may contribute to findings of liability. Examples include misspelled words such as "mussels" (for muscles) and uteriss (for uterus).

Always have readily available both a medical and standard dictionary for reference when writing patient care and related documentation. Clinical managers and facility/system administrators should also consider developing lists of lay and medical terms that are frequently misspelled and disseminating them to staff for training use.

Regarding extraneous verbiage not affecting patient care, a basic rule of thumb to remember is that information related only to patient examination, evaluation, diagnosis, prognosis, or intervention belongs in a patient care record. As an example, it would be wholly appropriate to record in the subjective portion of a SOAP note a patient's verbalization of his or her pain symptoms. It would be inappropriate to comment in the record irrelevant information about another health care provider's demeanor during official exchange about patient care (e.g., "Mar. 12, 200x/0400: Called Dr. Smith regarding patient's c/o stomachache. Dr. Smith *seemed irritated about receiving the call, but* ordered Maalox for the patient p.r.n.-Regina Doe, RN") (italicized material to be deleted).

Documentation Problems: Physician Orders: Transcription Problems; Examining and Intervening on Behalf of Patients Without Written Orders

Nurses and nurse practitioners, physician assistants, physical, occupational, and speech therapists, and other primary health care providers working in either inpatient or ambulatory care settings who read doctors' and other referring providers' preprinted or typed orders normally have no difficulty interpreting their meaning; however, handwritten orders written in haste—particularly during emergency situations—are often illegible. Health care professionals caring for patients pursuant to such referrals must be sure to clarify any ambiguities before carrying out orders, rather than making possibly erroneous assumptions about what is meant, to prevent patient injuries and potentially compensable events that could ripen into legal actions for health care malpractice.

Facility and departmental managers must establish policies that encourage providers who interpret physicians' orders to seek clarification of orders that appear ambiguous. These policies should be in writing and should be disseminated to all providers covered by their provisions. The policies should delineate appropriate methods for questioning such orders and spell out acceptable procedures for challenging suspected erroneous orders. Providers should remember to document carefully their inquiries and physician responses regarding ambiguities in diagnostic and treatment orders.

State law, facility policy, accreditation standards, and local custom govern the practice of caring for patients under verbal versus written physician's orders. Referral orders involving referring providers and consultants also raise important documentation issues. For most health care providers, the law requires written referral orders to treat patients referred by physicians and others for care. Even when allowed by law, clinicians such as physical therapists in direct access states who evaluate patients under verbal referral orders should always require the referring physician, dentist, or other provider to authenticate such orders expeditiously with signed written orders to enhance communication and protect both the referring provider and the clinician to whom the patient is referred. A sample form letter for requesting such orders appears in Exhibit 5–2.

Exhibit 5-2   Sample Request for Written Referral Orders to Accompany Verbal Referral Orders

Anytown Community Hospital, Anytown, USA Physical Therapy Clinic

May 1, 200x
To: Dr. Doe
From: Reginald P. Hasenfus, PT
Subject: Written referral orders re Patient dx

Dear Dr. Doe:

Please sign the enclosed referral order and return it to me in the enclosed stamped envelope so that we may complete our records and commence patient intervention for Mr. Tom Smith. Per your request during our telephonic consultation of April 29, 200x, I have examined Mr. Smith. I am enclosing the report of my examination, evaluative findings, and physical therapy diagnosis. Thank you for your prompt response.

Sincerely,

Reginald P. Hasenfus, PT
Chief Physical Therapist

Documentation Error: Untimely Documentation of Patient Care Activities

No factor contributes more to effective communication among health care providers simultaneously caring for patients than does the timely documentation of care. Failure to timely document important patient clinical information that other providers can use to prevent or alleviate patient suffering or to effect speedier recovery or optimal function is a form of professional negligence.

Ideally, timely documentation of patient care occurs concurrently with the rendition of care. In reality, however, patient care notation is often made at the end of a work shift. The further in time documentation of care occurs from the actual rendition of care or observation of a significant patient event or condition, the less accurate it becomes.

Attorneys examining health care providers in depositions or at trial often successfully challenge the accuracy of their documentation of patient care based on untimely notation. They persuasively argue before juries and judges that a provider's memory of critical events—like that of any percipient witness to an event—fades with the passage of time. Notation of care or patient status made hours, days, or even weeks after the fact, then, is less credible than when it is documented contemporaneously with care or observation.

Equally untimely as documentation made too long after care is rendered is documentation that is made before care is actually rendered. Consider, for example, the following hypothetical situation:

> A, a clinical physical therapist at ABC General Hospital, examines patient B for a complaint of interscapular myofascial pain. As part of her plan of care, A initiates moist heat, myofascial mobilization, ultrasound, and active range of motion exercises for patient B. Before patient B is finished with her first treatment session, A completes his initial patient care note, stating in part that "B had no adverse reaction to the initial treatment." Several minutes later, C, A's physical therapist assistant, informs A that B sustained a skin burn from the moist heat treatment. To correct his initial misimpression of patient B's tolerance of treatment, A must then either write an addendum to his original note or cross out and correct the erroneous portion of the original note. In either case, A's credibility is diminished, and if the incident devolves into a lawsuit, a jury or judge would probably be less likely generally to believe A's testimony about patient B's care than if the erroneous comment about patient B's status had not been improperly and incorrectly written in advance.

The physical therapist in this example could have prevented the loss of credibility regarding his testimony about patient B's overall care by having waited until patient B completed her initial treatment session to document her postintervention status.

Occasionally, providers will be required to document entries that are made some time after care has been rendered or after important information about a patient's status has already been observed. Such a late entry may necessarily occur when the provider may not have ready access to the patient's record or, as in the previous hypothetical situation, when additional clinically pertinent information about the patient becomes available only after the initial note is completed. A late entry should always be labeled as an "addendum" or "follow-on entry" to avoid a later inference that spoliation, or improper alteration of the patient's record, occurred. Also, a late entry should be labeled with the date and time that it is written. If a late entry does not build on the entry immediately preceding it, then some reference to the prior entry being amended must be made in the body of the late entry.

An example of how to document correctly the original and late entries illustrated in the hypothetical situation mentioned previously appears in Exhibit 5–3.

Exhibit 5–3   Example of Documenting a Necessary Late Patient Care Entry

ABC General Hospital Physical Therapy Department
Oct. 31, 200x

S: 49 y o F, dx: right interscapular myofascial pain syndrome, referred by Dr. Johansen of Pain Clinic for "evaluation and appropriate treatment." Hx of R FOOSH Oct. 20, 200x. No fx in RUE, acc to x-ray report in pt.'s OPR, dtd. Oct. 21, 200x. Pt. rates her localized pain (see diagram) as 6/10 and constant. No rad, neg. sensory sx, acc to pt. Meds: Motrin, Robaxin. Neg. prior hx. Pt. is homemaker and avocational painter.

O: GMT NL, BUE. FAROM BUE and C sp. Reflexes 2+/symm., BUE. SLT intact BUE and C & T sp. Neg. deformity; 12 trigger points of pain along sup. and med. R scapular border. Posture NL.

A: Myofascial pain syndrome, R interscapular region, secondary to R upper quarter trauma 10 days ago. ADL dysfunction (homemaking and painting activities).

P: MH, US, myofascial mobilization, AROM B Scapula and C & T sp., in clinic × 5. Pt. verbalizes decreased local sx. From 6/10 to 4/10 p/ initial rx. No adverse reaction to rx.

G: Decrease pain sx to 0–1/10 × 2–3 wks, so that pt. can carry out 1 pain-free ADL; prevent recurrence through pt. education.

ADDENDUM: Oct. 31, 200x/1400: Initial entry of this date incorrectly stated that pt. had no adverse reaction to initial care. Approx. 5 min. subsequent to note being written at 1330, pt. reportedly sustained a skin burn from MH over R medial scapular border, as reported to me by Carl Modality, PTA. Burn appears bright red, painful, small 2" diam. unbroken blister. I called Dr. Johansen and reported findings; pt. treated w/ice pack × 20 min, per Dr. Johansen VO. Pain and redness completely resolved. F/U w/ Dr. Johansen in a.m. or p.r.n. earlier.—Bob Therapist, PT.

Documentation Error: Identifying the Filing of an Incident Report in the Patient Care Record

Patient, visitor, and staff injuries unfortunately will occur from time to time in health care settings, regardless of precautions taken by clinical managers, clinicians, and support staff. When such nosocomial injuries occur, careful objective documentation of information that the provider writing about the injury perceives is critically important. Careful, complete documentation of an injury serves at least three purposes: to promote optimal quality care to the injured party, to serve the risk management function of protecting the facility from unwarranted liability exposure, and to form the basis for further training of staff members to try to prevent similar incidents in the future.

Whenever any adverse event involving actual or potential injury to a patient, visitor, or staff member occurs, a formal incident report should be completed and forwarded through the clinical manager to a centralized risk management office for review and retention. An incident report also must be completed whenever a medication error occurs or when a patient or visitor makes a formal complaint about a facility, system, or its staff.

Administrators and clinical managers should educate their staffs that the completion of an incident report under such circumstances is the norm and will not, in and of itself, constitute a stigma against any provider potentially responsible for an adverse event. Staff members should also be educated as to why an incident report is so critically important. Because memories fade relatively quickly after an event is perceived, it is vital to document right away what happened to an injured party.

Writers of these reports, clinical managers, and facility/system administrators can feel secure in knowing that incident reports, like other quality assurance/improvement/management or attorney-work product documents, normally enjoy qualified immunity from release to patients, their attorneys, and others seeking to obtain them. Because incident reports necessarily contain more detailed administrative information than a concomitant patient care note concerning care rendered to an injured party, however, they should not be filed in the injured party's patient care record.

Also, to avoid drawing a patient or attorney's attention to the fact that an incident report has been filed, providers must be careful not to mention in the patient care record that an incident report has been filed. This precaution is not advocating "hiding the ball." Documentation of the existence of an incident report has no place in a patient care record because an incident report contains purely administrative and not clinical information.

Documentation Problem: Failing to Delineate Patient Care Rendered or Identify Clinical Information Supplied by Another Provider

Not every observation or finding described by a clinician in a patient examination, evaluation, or intervention note concerns observations or findings that the clinician perceived firsthand. Very often, other health care professionals, support staff, and other persons supply clinically pertinent information about a patient that is incorporated into primary documentation of care. Patient care carried out by another provider, as well as clinical information supplied by another person to the writer of a patient care note, should be clearly attributed to the source person.

Failure to denote another person's responsibility for clinical information supplied to the writer of a patient care note may result in legal responsibility being ascribed exclusively to the note writer for the information at issue. This may be the case even when the information clearly could not have emanated from the writer, for example, where a surgeon or radiologist furnishes information about a patient's medical status to a nurse, physical or occupational therapist, or other nonphysician provider caring for the patient.

Consider the following hypothetical case:

> X, a staff occupational therapist at Anytown General Hospital, conducts an initial musculoskeletal evaluation of patient P, pursuant to a proper written order from Dr. Z. Patient P's diagnosis is right carpal tunnel syndrome, status-postcarpal tunnel release 7 days ago. Patient P is referred for "evaluation and appropriate exercises." During her evaluation of patient P, X telephones Dr. Z for consultation, after patient P reveals to X that she fell onto her outstretched right hand 2 days postoperatively and is now experiencing local sharp pain at the proximal thenar eminence. X suspects a carpal fracture. Patient P's chart contains no information about recent right wrist radiographs. Dr. Z advises X that she just examined patient P yesterday and ordered x-rays of her right wrist, which were negative. Dr. Z tells X to proceed with postoperative range of motion exercises. X documents in her evaluation note that patient P's right wrist x-rays were normal, without ascribing responsibility for the information to Dr. Z. X also fails to document Dr. Z's verbal instructions to her to proceed with treatment. X proceeds with treatment, which consists of home active exercises. On her 1-week recheck, patient P's right proximal wrist pain has increased significantly, and she is tender to palpation over the scaphoid bone. X walks to the radiology department, where she reviews patient P's prior right wrist x-rays with Dr. R, a radiology resident. Dr. R had just officially read patient P's x-rays and documented the results 2 days ago; they show a scaphoid fracture. When X reveals this finding to patient P, patient P becomes infuriated with X over the erroneous prior reading of her radiograph and threatens to sue. Even though Dr. Z most probably will concede that he misread patient P's radiographs and communicated to X that they were normal, an

ambiguity still exists in X's initial evaluation note, in which it appears that X personally read patient P's radiographs as normal. This misinterpretation of X's evaluation note could have easily been prevented had X documented patient P's radiographic findings in the objective section of her note as follows: "X-rays of R wrist taken Mar. 19, 200x, by Dr. Z and read as normal. (Information obtained telephonically from Dr. Z on Mar. 20, 200x)." The following phrase should also have appeared in the assessment portion of X's initial note: "P cleared by Dr. Z for active range of motion exercises."

Similar misinterpretations over who is responsible for patient care or diagnostic information can also occur when assistants, aides, residents, interns, and students on clinical affiliations relate clinical information to providers who are privileged to document in patient care records and the writer fails to denote who actually provided the care or furnished the information.

For example, consider the following hypothetical situation:

A physical therapist assistant administering therapeutic exercises to a rehabilitation patient relates to the supervising physical therapist that the patient displayed anterior shoulder pain during active arm exercises. The proper course of action for the supervising physical therapist (who is not present at the scene) is to annotate that finding in a progress note and credit the physical therapist assistant as the source of the information. Such a note might appear as follows:

Dec. 23, 200x/1900 P: 67 y o M, dx: s/p R CVA w/ residual L UE weakness.

S: Shawn Jones, PTA, reported telephonically that pt. c/o increased L ant. shoulder pain with PNF; no apparent subluxation, swelling, or other objective signs reported. I was at another location. Directed Mr. Jones to d/c exercises for now and instruct pt. and wife to cont. w/ MH or CP, according to pt. preference, p.r.n.

P: Will re-examine pt. this p.m. for new L UE pain complaint.—Philomena Therapist, PT

Whenever a primary health care provider receives and documents clinical information about an adverse change in a patient's condition derived from another professional or support person, the primary provider becomes obligated to re-examine the patient expeditiously or risk professional negligence-based health care malpractice liability exposure for patient injuries for the negligent failure to appropriately monitor the patient.

Documentation Error: Blaming or Disparaging Another Provider in the Patient Care Record

Information that disparages another health care provider or blames any provider for a patient's condition either expressly or by implication has no place in the patient care record. Such information has no clinical relevance to patient care. One type of entry often seen in patient care records that has an implication of blame is notation that documents missed patient appointments.

Consider the following hypothetical situation:

> Patient Y underwent an arthroscopic debridement and repair of her torn left medial meniscus yesterday. At ABC Hospital, post-operative arthroscopic knee procedure patients go to physical therapy 1 day preoperatively for preoperative examination and patient education about the postoperative exercise program. In this case, a miscommunication between the orthopedic ward and physical therapy prevented patient Y from being seen preoperatively. Although all three providers involved—the orthopedic surgeon, the charge nurse for the orthopedic ward, and the orthopedic physical therapist—could give in to the temptation to document patient Y's missed preoperative physical therapy appointment defensively, it would be unproductive and perhaps inaccurate to cast aspersions on each other for the mistake. Examples of inappropriate entries in this case would include the following three examples:

Example 1: Apr. 1, 200x/1400

P: One-day post-op L arthroscopic medial meniscus debridement and repair.

S: Minimal swelling; no drainage. Pt. reluctant to do isometric quadriceps sets. PT neglected to see pt. for pre-op teaching.

P: To PT today for post-op rehab per protocol.

G: D/C crutches in 1 wk; FFAROM L knee × 2–4 wks; 1 pain-free ADL × 6–8 wks.—Otto Ortho, M.D.

Example 2: Apr. 1, 200x/1500

S: 32 y o M, computer programmer, s/p L arthroscopic medial meniscus debridement and repair yesterday. To clinic via w/c. Referred for post-op rehab per protocol. Meds: Tylenol p.r.n. (none since 11 a.m. today).

O: Alert; seems disturbed over his missed app't for pre-op education. In bulky dressing; removed; no drainage. AAROM, L knee: 0/65 degrees; min. swelling. N/V intact. Rest of LQ screen WNL.

A: s/p L arthroscopic medial meniscus debridement and repair yesterday. Ready for post-op rehab; crutch walking PWB (50%). Note: Missed pre-op app't was due to the ward failing to send down a preop consult.

P: CW today, begin QS, SLR, AAROM; progress per protocol. Pt. is I on crutches, at approximately 50% PWB, level and stairs; understood and safely carried out all instructed activities.

STG: D/C crutches in 1 wk; FFAROM L knee × 2–4 wks.

LTG: 1 pain-free ADL × 6–8 wks.—Ron Therapist, PT

Example 3: Apr. 1, 200x/1415

P: One-day post-op L arthroscopic medial meniscus debridement and repair.

S: Dr. Ortho just ordered pt. to PT today for post-op rehab. Pt. visibly upset p/ Dr. visit because of missed pre-op PT eval. app't. It was my fault that pt. didn't get to PT pre-op. I saw Dr. Ortho's standing pre-op order but forgot to send pt. to PT because I was involved w/six other admissions. Sorry!

P: To PT now in w/c for post-op rehab and crutch gait trg. PWB (50%) per protocol.

G: I CW PWB X 1 day; I pain management; prevent wound infection; return to work sx-free.—Regina Smith, RN

These three hypothetical patient care notes illustrate several important points. Dr. Ortho should not have displayed his anger over the missed preoperative teaching appointment in front of the patient. He also should not have documented in his progress note that the physical therapist was negligent in failing to see the patient preoperatively. (This conjecture was, in fact, inaccurate.)

Dr. Ortho's reaction to the patient's missed appointment and the documentation of his speculation as to its cause started a chain reaction of patient dissatisfaction and defensive documentation by other providers on the team that was irrelevant, disruptive to patient care, and unproductive. The end result may be (depending on the outcomes of this patient's care) that the patient files a complaint, claim, or even a legal and/or administrative action because of what occurred. If that would occur, then the defensive documentation illustrated previously here would be very helpful in support of the patient's health care malpractice case.

Just as Dr. Ortho and Mr. Therapist should not have blamed physical therapy and nursing, respectively, for the missed appointment in the patient's care record, Ms. Smith should not have conceded blame for the incident in the patient's record. Again, her admission has no clinical relevance and therefore no place in the patient care record.

Problems of this type are best addressed informally between members of the patient care team in the setting of an interdisciplinary quality management committee meeting. The focus of such a meeting is primarily on how to resolve the problem, not on targeting individuals. If more formal action is required, then the surgeon or another team member should initiate an incident report, wherein reasons for the missed appointment can be more freely detailed. Of course, an incident report would be required if the patient suffered injury as a result of the missed appointment. The incident report, as a quality assurance/improvement or attorney work-product document, is normally immune from release to the patient or the patient's attorney under state or federal law.

Even in an incident report, however, a provider is not free to defame another provider by making a false accusation that damages the defamed provider's professional reputation in the eyes of others in the relevant health care community. Purely personal defamatory remarks are legally actionable as intentional torts (wrongs).

Defamation has two varieties: libel and slander. Written defamatory remarks about another provider, such as might appear in a patient care record, incident report, or other document, constitute *libel*. Also included within the definition of libel are defamatory statements made on computer, videotape, or other relatively permanent media. Spoken defamation is called *slander*. If a defendant is found liable for defamation, then the damages might include not only compensatory money damages for loss of the victim's personal and professional reputation, but also punitive, or

> *Defamation* is a communication to a third party of an untrue statement about a person that damages the defamed person's good reputation in the community. Although normally a person claiming to be defamed must prove any losses suffered as a result of the defamation, damages may be presumed and may not need to be proven for victims who are professionals and business persons. The two classifications of defamation are as follows:
>
> - *Slander*: oral defamation
> - *Libel*: written, pictoral, and other more permanent modes of defamation

exemplary, damages intended to punish a wrongdoer. In many states, the defendant may be personally responsible for payment of the judgment in such a case, where the defendant's insurer is statutorily relieved of responsibility for indemnification for judgments involving malicious intentional torts and/or punitive damages.

Documentation Error: Expressing Personal Feelings about a Patient or Patient Family Member or Significant Other in the Patient Care Record

Just as patient care documentation entries can disparage health care providers, inappropriate statements written about patients in their records may also constitute actionable defamation. Health care providers documenting patient examinations, evaluations, or interventions must exercise special caution to avoid making inappropriate personal comments about patients under their care. For example, (actual observed) attributions such as "malingerer," "supra tentorial symptoms," "manipulator," and "pseudointellectual" are all inappropriate. Such comments, if discovered by the patient, will justifiably sour the patient–professional relationship and make the patient more litigation prone for health care malpractice and defamation causes of action. In such a case, the health care provider will be in the nearly impossible position of trying to establish at trial during the defense case that the documentation in issue accurately characterized the patient.

Despite the fear of a defamation action, a health care provider is ethically obligated to document findings that negate a patient's assertions of symptoms. This, however, must be done very carefully. Statements such as "objective examination normal" and "palpation, even to light skin touch, results in severe pain response by patient" are, if accurate, appropriate. More risky, but perhaps still appropriate, comments are ones such as evaluative conclusions that state "rule out subjective exaggeration of symptoms, based on normal objective findings" and "rule out secondary gain." Conclusions based on conjecture, such as "objective findings do not justify subjective complaints," are inappropriate and dangerous and must be avoided.

Providers must also be vigilant when they transcribe statements made by patients during examinations and interventions. Any statement made by a patient that is documented in the patient care record must appear in quotation marks. For example, if a patient says to a physical therapist during an examination for a complaint of work-related low back pain that his back does not hurt him now, then the therapist should quote the patient, rather than paraphrase the patient's remark, in the subjective section of the evaluation note. When documenting such a statement that is clearly contrary to the patient's self-interest, the provider should have the patient confirm the statement before writing it in the patient care record. Although it may seem to be defensive health care, consider having a witness present when the patient confirms such a statement. Ethically, however, such a statement requires documentation in the patient care record because it is clinically pertinent information about the patient.

In the rare case in which a patient plainly asserts that he or she is falsifying symptoms (i.e., committing fraud) to bolster a legal case or to dupe an insurance company or workers' compensation board, the provider should immediately report that finding to his or her supervisor, organizational administrator, or legal counsel for further action.

Documentation Suggestion: Document Observations and Findings Objectively

Subjective information belongs exclusively in the subjective ("S") section of a patient care note. Clinical information documented in other sections of the note ("O," "A," and "P") must be written in objective, unambiguous, and, to the extent possible, quantifiable terms to promote clear, effective communication with other providers. Providers should avoid documenting ambiguous conclusions about a patient's status, such as "appears within normal limits," "apparent muscle tightness," and "tolerated treatment well," as well as ambiguous intervention plans, such as "routine strengthening exercises" and "conservative measures."

Documentation Suggestion: Document With Specificity

Similar to clinical information that is ambiguous and lacks objectivity is information that lacks specificity. When generalizations are made or when information that clearly can and should be quantified is not, providers miss an important opportunity to communicate effectively about their patients to other providers.

For example, if an occupational therapist conducting two-point discrimination sensory testing of a patient's hand writes "within normal limits," then other providers reading the findings can only guess at their meaning. The preferred way of documenting such findings would be to quantify in standard terms (here, millimeters) the patient's discrimination of two static or moving sharp points and report results (pictorially and numerically) for specific locations on specific fingers.

Another example concerns a hypothetical physician's assistant conducting reflex testing of a patient during a neurologic examination. If the physician assistant reports "reflexes WNL," then other providers reading the note have no clue as to which reflexes were tested or what "WNL" means. More specific and meaningful would be the following report: "biceps, triceps, and brachioradialis reflexes 2+/symmetrical/brisk in both upper limbs."

Documentation Error: Recording *Hearsay* (Second-Hand Information) as If It Were Fact

Documenting hearsay as if it were fact is a common and dangerous practice that can leave health care providers in a position of increased vulnerability to health care malpractice and defamation liability exposure. Hearsay is a legal term of art used to describe any extrajudicial (out-of-court) statement offered as evidence in court for the truth of the matter asserted in it. Regarding patient care documentation, hearsay describes a statement made by one person and adopted as fact by another person. That is, hearsay describes second-hand input.

Take, for example, the case in which a physical therapist, P, who intervenes for patients bedside on hospital wards, enters patient Q's room. Q is a 65-year-old male patient whose status is post left cerebrovascular accident, with right hemiparesis and poor standing balance. Q is not yet ambulatory. On entering Q's room, P notices Q lying on the floor next to his bed, moaning. The bed rail is down. Sitting on a chair next to the bed is Q's wife, R. When P asks R what happened, she replies, "The bed rail was down, and he rolled out of bed." P calls loudly for help; Q is examined by Dr. S and found to be unhurt, except for two minor bruises on his right elbow and right femoral greater trochanter. Q's status would be correctly described in progress notes by P and Dr. S as follows:

June 25, 200x/1425

P: L CVA; R hemiparesis; bedside PT pt.

S: Found lying on floor next to bed. Dr. S examined pt. and stated pt. is "fine, except for two small bruises, one on R elbow, one on R greater trochanter." Dr. S ordered PT held for today.

P: Hold PT today, recheck status in a.m.

G: Progress to standing × 1 wk—Endie Tee, PT

June 25, 200x/1428

P: L CVA; R hemiparesis.

S: Mr. Tee, PT, reported that pt. found on floor next to bed. Examination WNL, except for 2 small bruises, one on R elbow, one on R greater trochanter.

P: Hold PT for today; monitor V/S q 4 hrs × 24 hrs. Re-examine in a.m.—Vigil Lant, MD

Each provider only documented as firsthand the clinical information that he personally perceived. The physical therapist and physician each correctly attributed hearsay information provided by the other appropriately in his note. Also, neither provider made mention in patient care documentation of how patient Q might have alighted from his bed. That information was correctly excluded from their documentation. Such information should instead be documented in an incident report. Because Q's wife supplied that information, her hearsay statements must be appropriately recorded in the incident report.

Another example of hearsay involves information related by a patient presenting for examination with incomplete prior documentation of the patient's status. Consider, for instance, the case in which a physical therapist is examining a patient pursuant to a written physician referral, with a diagnosis of left lateral (humeral) epicondylitis. The therapist does not have any reports about radiographs. The patient volunteers that the referring physician took radiographs of the left elbow and read them as normal. If the therapist relies on that information in his or her examination, evaluation, and diagnosis, it must be properly attributed to the patient as the source of the information. It would, therefore, be incorrect for the therapist to write "x-ray WNL" as part of the examination. Instead, the therapist would correctly document in his or her patient care notation as follows, including reference to the patient as a source for information about the left elbow x-ray and the patient's allergic status:

Aug. 5, 200x

S: 45 y o F, dx: L lat. epicondylitis; referred for "evaluation and appropriate rx."

O: Alert, cooperative. FAROM BUE; GMT NL BUE. Neg. swelling peri-L lat. epicondyle. SLT intact BUE. Min. TTP L proximal lat. epicondyle. Mod. c/o pain L lat. epicondyle w/resisted L wrist extension and passive L wrist flexion. Per pt., x-ray of L elbow, taken by Dr. X, Aug. 3, 200x, reported to her as WNL by Dr. X. (No report available; Dr. X and staff on vacation.)

A: L lat. epicondylitis.

P: HCP × 5 (pt. reports "no allergy to HC"); gentle AROM, progress to PREs. No objective signs, or patient complaint of problems, with rx.

G: Decrease sx 25% × 2 wks; I pain-free ADL (cooking, tennis) × 2–4 wks; prevent recurrence through ADL hints.—John P. Doe, PT

Documentation Suggestion: Exercise Special Caution When Countersigning Another Provider's, Student's, or Intern's Patient Care Notation

Staff physicians, clinical preceptors, and other primary health care providers are frequently called on to serve as clinical instructors for health professions students. In that role, providers routinely countersign patient care notations made by students under their supervision. In most cases, such authentication is required to make the student's documentation legally acceptable.

> Once countersigned, a student or intern's patient care note is legally adopted by the supervising health care professional as his or her own note. The preceptor then shares legal responsibility for what is written therein.

Providers who countersign another persons' patient care notes are urged to proofread carefully what is written, because, like a guarantor who cosigns for a loan for another person, the countersigning health care professional assumes legal responsibility for the information contained in the note.

If the supervising clinical instructor or mentor observes incomplete or inaccurate information in a student or intern's patient care note, then the supervisor is obligated to correct the note before signing it. This may be done by having the student correct discrepancies in the documentation or, as supervisor, by correcting the note and initialing the modifications made. Once countersigned, a student or intern's patient care note is legally adopted by the supervising health care professional as his or her own note. The preceptor then shares legal responsibility for what is written therein.

Documentation Error: Failure to Document a Patient's Informed Consent to Examination and Intervention

The concept of informed consent recognizes the fundamental human rights principle that every adult patient with full mental capacity has the right of control over health care decision making and must be given sufficient clinical disclosure information by a health care provider to make an informed choice. For many procedures, such as surgical procedures and administration of anesthesia, state statutory law spells out documentation requirements that serve as legally sufficient evidence of a patient's informed consent to intervention. For most routine health care interventions, however, there are no statutory formats to comply with to document patients' informed consent. Providers, therefore, should consider devising their own formats for documenting patients' informed consent to routine health care interventions.

Documentation Suggestion: Document Thoroughly Patient/Family/Significant Other Understanding of and Safe Compliance with Discharge, Home Care, and Follow-Up Instructions

In a managed care environment, characterized by diminished reimbursement for health care services, the legal standards of care for physicians; nurses; physical, occupational, and speech therapists; orthotists and prosthetists; and other health care providers include the issuance of written home care instructions to patients on discharge from the hospital or from outpatient care. Providers are urged to retain master copies of standardized home care instructions given routinely to patients and/or families/significant others caring for patients at home. These forms should be an integral part of a clinic procedures manual.

Service chiefs and risk managers should ensure that staff clinicians provide written, personalized home care instructions to every patient. If issuance of these written home care instructions becomes a standard clinical practice, then even in the absence of documentation of their issuance, providers testifying at a health care malpractice trial years after their issuance can truthfully testify that the issuance of written home care instructions is a universal and customary practice. Such evidence of customary practice, even when the provider cannot recall a specific case or patient, is usually admissible as substantive evidence of compliance with the custom in an individual case.

As with informed consent, a provider should document that a patient and/or family member or significant other understands, safely carries out, and accepts responsibility for compliance with a home program of care.

Documentation of home care/follow-up instructions issued to a patient/family member/significant other responsible for home care on discharge

Required elements:

- Written home care instructions issued

- Patient/family member/significant other advised about any special precautions or limitations associated with the home care program

- Instructions for follow-up re-examination, as indicated

- Written documentation that patient/family member/significant other understands and consents to the home care program, acknowledges responsibility for compliance with it, and demonstrates the ability to carry it out competently and safely

> It may constitute patient abandonment to not offer necessary follow-up to a home care patient.

The provider should also document any special precautions or limitations on the patient's activities, as well as follow-up care instructions. It may constitute patient abandonment to not offer necessary follow-up to a home care patient.

Such documentation in a patient discharge note might appear as follows in the Problem-Status-Plan (P-S-P) format:

Oct. 31, 200x

P: L CVA, R UE hemiparesis.

S: Alert, cooperative; independent in all relevant ADL; FAROM w/NL GMT BUE. SLT intact BUE. Reflexes 2+/symm. BUE. Normal R UE proprioception.

P: Discharge to home. Written instructions for home exercises, including PNF and AROM exercises, issued to pt. Pt. to stop program if severe pain, swelling, or loss of sensation occurs and report symptoms to me immediately. Pt. understands all, agrees to comply with program as outlined in handout, and safely demonstrated all recommended home exercises. F/U 2–3 wks or p.r.n.

G: Increase R UE strength to enable pt. to perform prestroke household duties within 1–2 mos.—J. Ray, OTR/L

Documentation Suggestion: Carefully Document a Patient's Noncompliance with Provider Directives or Orders

Documenting patients' noncompliance with care is an important risk-management tool to protect health care providers individually and their employing health care organizations from health care malpractice liability in the event that a claim or lawsuit ensues, resulting from alleged injuries incident to care. Providers should carefully document noncompliance events involving patients under their care, such as refusal to comply with the facility's "no-smoking" policy or comply with dietary restrictions, refusal to ask for ambulatory assistance where the patient cannot ambulate independently (with or without assistive devices), refusal to use ambulatory assistive devices when ordered, and refusal to take medications as ordered or to carry out exercises or other important interventions. Careful, thorough, objective, nondefensive documentation, including specific therapeutic orders violated and dates, times, and circumstances of patient noncompliance, should be included in such notation.

Documentation Suggestion: Carefully Document a Patient's or Family Member's/Significant Other's Possible Contributory Negligence Related to Alleged Patient Injuries or Lack of Progress

In some instances, health professional negligence can be inferred or presumed if patients are injured under circumstances in which they normally would not suffer injury, absent a provider's probable negligence. Such circumstances might include patient falls while transferring or ambulating, falling from the bed onto the floor, medication overdoses, burns while under heat or ice treatment, and tissue ischemia from tight compression garments, casts, or orthoses.

Under the legal concept of *res ipsa loquitur*, professional negligence might be presumed against a health care provider in the previously mentioned situations unless there is documented evidence that the patient or a family member/significant other caused or contributed to the patient's injuries. Like everyone, a patient can be contributorily negligent (i.e., fail to conform to the standards required by law for his or her own safety and protection from harm).

Health care providers must carefully document a patient's refusal to comply with recommendations and instructions, as well as a patient's misuse or tampering with exercise equipment or other therapeutic devices, such as electric heating pads or neuromuscular stimulation devices. When a patient is contributorily negligent and suffers injury as a result, the patient cannot normally invoke *res ipsa loquitur* as an aid to proving a case of health care malpractice.

> The end result of a carefully designed documentation program is optimal quality patient care.

QUESTIONS AND CASES FOR STUDY

1. A is a student physical therapist assistant who is about to graduate from her entry-level education program in a large metropolitan area. She sends out over 175 "canned" resumes and "to whom it may concern" cover letters to prospective employers. After 6 weeks, A has only one response—a rejection. What was wrong about A's approach to health professional job-seeking? How would you do it differently?

2. Cite an example from past experience of organizational culture. What things did members of the organization do to share common beliefs and values and attempt to bond? How did you view these manifestations of shared beliefs and values?

3. Look back at Rooke and Torbert's continuum of leadership. What kind of leader is the best fit for surgical team in a large medical

center? Which type is best for a physical rehabilitation team in the same medical center?

4. *Working Woman* magazine's annual comparative salary survey consistently reveals disparities in compensation between women and men doing the same work, particularly in health care service delivery. What factors contribute to this phenomenon? What would you do as a business leader to help end such gender discrimination?

5. Consider the workplace stressors that affect you personally. List them in descending order of intensity. Devise and list strategies (game plans) and tactics (means to implement solutions) to address them. Put your remediation plans into effect immediately.

REFERENCES, READINGS, AND RESOURCES

1. Barada PW. Before you go. *HRMagazine*. 1998;43:99–102.

2. Berglas S. Chronic time abuse. *Harvard Business Review*. June 2004, 90–97.

3. Bernhard B. Shaping up: Some employers now offering incentives to stay healthy. *San Antonio Express News*. Jan. 22, 2006, 6N.

4. Blount E. M.D.s who mind their P's and Q's shouldn't misplace their modifiers. *Wall Street Journal*. Jan. 27, 1999, B1.

5. Bosman J. Stuck at the edges of the ad game: Women feel sidelined in subtle ways. *New York Times*. Nov. 22, 2005, C1, 5.

6. Brounstein M. *Managing Teams for Dummies*. Indianapolis, IN: John Wiley and Sons, 2000.

7. Brooks ML. *Exploring Medical Language*, 4th ed. St. Louis: Mosby Year-book, Inc., 1998.

8. Challenger JE. Changing careers can be hazardous to worklife. *San Antonio Express News*. Apr. 9, 2006, 2M.

9. Challenger JE. Let prospective employer set interview agenda. *San Antonio Express News*. Feb. 19, 2006, 2N.

10. Clifton DW. *Physical Rehabilitation's Role in Disability Management: Unique Perspectives for Success*. Philadelphia: Elsevier, 2004.

11. Coping with work-related stress. *San Antonio Express News*. April 23, 2006, 8S.

12. Ertel D. Getting past yes: Negotiating as if implementation mattered. *Harvard Business Review*. 2004;82:60–68.

13. Fandray D. Getting things done. *Continental Magazine*. Oct. 2005, 86–88.

14. Farmer J. Hiring staff in private practice. *PT Magazine*. Sept. 2004, 46–49.

15. Fisher R, Ury W, Patton B. *Getting to Yes*. London: Penguin Books, 2001.

16. Fleck C. Make the most of your experience. *AARP Bulletin*. Jan. 2006, 18–19.

17. Goodman CK. Reverse mentoring now a workplace fact. *San Antonio Express News*. May 7, 2006, 2G.

18. Grensing-Pophal L. Motivate managers to review performance. *HR Magazine.* Mar. 2001, 44–48.

19. Jeffrey C. The watched: Who's zooming in on whom? *Mother Jones.* 2005;30:26–27.

20. Kallick R. The resume: An effective document increases job possibilities. *Health Careers Today.* Feb. 2005, 6, 15.

21. Kettenbach G. *Writing SOAP Notes,* 3rd ed. Philadelphia: FA Davis Co., 2004.

22. Kinsman M. Workplace success often tied to social intelligence. *San Antonio Express News.* May 21, 2006, 10R, 14N.

23. Kinsman M. The job interview dreaded by many. *San Antonio Express News.* Apr. 23, 2006, 10R, 12R.

24. Kollenberg LO. Payment depends on documentation. *Biomechanics.* Feb. 1998, 39–43.

25. Kriemer S. Psychologists find new role in the workplace. *San Antonio Express News.* May 14, 2006, G2.

26. Kolb D, Williams J. Breakthrough bargaining. *Harvard Business Review.* Feb. 2001, 89–97.

27. Krueger AB. Job satisfaction is not just a matter of dollars. *New York Times.* Dec. 8, 2005, C3.

28. Lax DA, Sebenius JK. 3-D negotiation: Playing the whole game. *Harvard Business Review.* Nov. 2003, 65–72.

29. Lencioni P. *Death by Meeting.* San Francisco: Jossey-Bass, 2004.

30. Lohr S. How the game is played. *New York Times.* Dec. 5, 2005, C1, 8.

31. Lubin JS. Some do's and don'ts to help you hone your videoconferencing skills. *Wall Street Journal.* Feb. 7, 2006, B1.

32. Mausy A. Web conferencing: Smart tools for virtual meetings. *Texas Bar Journal.* Nov. 2003, 864.

33. McAtee DR III. Staying on top of your game. *Texas Bar Journal.* Feb. 2006, 142–143.

34. McIntyre MG. New boss means new expectations. *San Antonio Express News.* Apr. 16, 2006, G1.

35. Needleman SE. Be prepared when opportunity knocks. *Wall Street Journal.* Feb. 7, 2006, B3.

36. Nero ME. Temp agencies becoming permanent solution. *San Antonio Express News.* Jan. 22, 2006, 4N.

37. Orr C. How to make resume digitally friendly. *San Antonio Express News: Keys to Success.* Mar. 5, 2006, 3P.

38. Orr C. Women executives offer advice for success. *San Antonio Express News.* Feb. 19, 2006, 6N.

39. O'Shea D. How to get your foot in the door for interview. *San Antonio Express News.* Sept. 11, 2005, 3P.

40. Pavlik J. Working the office political machine. *Indianapolis Star.* Sept. 12, 2004, F7.

41. Pierson FM. *Principles and Techniques of Patient Care,* 2nd ed. Philadelphia: WB Saunders Co., 1998.

42. Quinn L, Gordon J. *Functional Outcomes Documentation for Rehabilitation.* St. Louis: Elsevier, 2003.

43. Resume revival: Simple ideas can pump new life into your job search. *San Antonio Express News: Career Focus.* Jan. 22, 2006, 2N.

44. Romanski E. Physicians beat burnout: Get a grip on stress before getting run down. *Humana's Your Practice.* Fall, 2004, 15.

45. Rooke D, Torbert WR. 7 transformations of leadership. *Harvard Business Review.* 2005;83:66–76.

46. Sakis JR, Kennedy DB. Violence at work. *Trial.* Dec. 2002, 32–36.

47. Scott RW. Manage stress so it doesn't manage you. *Risk Advisor.* Summer 2000, 1.

48. Scott RW. Incident reports: Protecting the record. *PT: Magazine of Physical Therapy.* 1996;4:24–25.

49. Stamer MH. *Functional Documentation.* Tucson, AZ: Therapy Skill Builders, 1995.

50. Talk show: Preparation key to success in interview. *San Antonio Express News.* Mar. 19, 2006, 4P.

51. Tapping hidden networks improves chances of landing job. *San Antonio Express News.* Apr. 23, 2006, 7R.

52. Thiruvengadam M. Sex, style and psychology. *San Antonio Express News.* Jan. 1, 2006, 1L.

53. Vanderwall S. Survey finds unscheduled absenteeism hitting seven-year high. *HRNews.* Nov. 1998, 14.

54. Working for a competitor likely in today's economy. *San Antonio Express News.* Apr. 9, 2006, 3M.

55. Yocum RF. *Documentation Skills for Quality Patient Care,* 2nd ed. Edwardsville, FL: Awareness Productions, 1999.

56. www.job-hunt.org (links to job websites)

The Future of Health Care Service Delivery Is in Your Hands

You are about to embark on a career journey that will keep you ever learning, excited, and satisfied for decades to come. Health care delivery and its allied administrative and clinical specialties really are special callings. In no other area of employment do providers routinely hold the lives and well-being of clients (patients) in their hands. You must accept the obligations associated with such responsibility, as well as the benefits and privileges thereunto appertaining. I know that you are ready to do so.

Health care is changing phenomenally, as employers, governments, insurers, and patients themselves all try to pare costs associated with care delivery; however, no matter what cost savings are realized over the next decade, the American health care system cannot continue to eat up more and more of the gross domestic product (GDP). At the current rate of growth of health expenditures, the system will consume $17 trillion, or 32% of GDP by 2030. No government can afford a health care system that costs so much.

The United States must have the courage to re-examine and implement a national health insurance system, probably managed by the federal government. As health care professionals charged to put patient interests first, we must endorse such a model sooner or later. We can mold the prospective model so that it creates a "win–win" outcome for all participants in the system.

At day's end, we will always be altruists who care about patients' welfare more than anything else. Health care professionals and organizations that espouse that business savvy is more important than altruism have lost their way. At the grassroots level, we still exist to serve our patients.

Why do we as health care professionals care so much about patients under our care? In part, we do so because we know that someday we and our family members will be patients who want the same caliber of care that we now deliver to strangers. Money is not everything. In fact, it is way behind what comes in first place—philanthropy. Answers.com defines philanthropy as "the effort to increase the well-being of humankind; love of humankind; and the promotion of human welfare." That is what we are all about. That is why you are entering this sacred profession. That is why the human race will survive and thrive.

Do well while doing good things for others. God bless you and let you prosper.

Sample Patient Rights and Responsibilities Document (Brooke Army Medical Center, San Antonio, Texas): English Version

Patients' Rights and Responsibilities
Brooke Army Medical Center
Fort Sam Houston, Texas

We at Brooke Army Medical Center (BAMC) hold the welfare and safety of the patient as our highest priority. The most important person in this medical center is you, our patient. Our goal is to provide you with the best medical care available. Our success will be reflected in your satisfaction with the treatment you receive. We regard your basic human rights with great importance. You have the right to freedom of expression, to make your own decisions, and to know that your human rights will be preserved and respected. The following is a list of patient rights and responsibilities.

Your Rights as a Patient

You have the right to receive respectful, considerate, and supportive treatment and service.

We will do our best to provide you with compassionate and respectful care at all times.

We will do everything possible to provide a safe hospital environment.

We will be attentive to your specific needs and requests, understanding that they should not interfere with medical care for you or for others.

We will not discriminate in providing you with care based on race, ethnicity, national origin, religion, gender, age, mental or physical disability, genetic information, sexual orientation, or source of payment.

You have the right to be involved in all aspects of your care.

We will make sure that you know which physician or care provider is primarily responsible for your care. We will explain the professional status and the role of persons who help in your care.

We will keep you fully informed about your condition, the results of tests we perform, and the treatment you receive.

We will clearly explain to you any treatments or procedures that we propose. We will request your written consent for procedures that carry more than minimal risk.

We will make sure that you are part of the decision-making process in your care. When there are dilemmas or differences over care decisions, we will include you in resolving them.

We will honor your right to refuse the care that we advise. (In some circumstances, especially for active duty patients, laws and regulations may override this right.)

We will honor your advance directive or medical power of attorney, regarding limits to the care that you wish to receive.

You have the right to receive timely and appropriate assessment and management of your pain.

We will routinely ask if you are suffering pain. If you are, we will evaluate it further and help you get relief.

You have the right to have your personal needs respected.

We will respect the confidentiality of your personal information throughout the institution. (For active duty persons, complete confidentiality may not be possible, based on requirements to report some conditions or findings.) We will respect your need for privacy in conversations, examinations, information sharing, and procedures. Also, you may request that a chaperone be present during an examination or procedure.

We will communicate with you in a language that you understand.

We will respect your need to feel safe and secure throughout the facility. Hospital employees will be identifiable with badges or nameplates.

We will take your concerns and complaints seriously and will work hard to resolve them.

We will respect your need for pastoral care and other spiritual services. Our chaplain service is on call at all times. Other spiritual support is welcome, as long as it does not interfere with patient care or hospital function.

We will respect your need to communicate with others, both family and friends. If it is medically necessary to limit your communications with others, we will tell you and your family why.

We will use soft fabric restraints, with close and frequent monitoring, if you become so confused that you are in danger of hurting yourself or others. We will untie the restraints as soon as we safely can do so.

You have the right to receive information on how to contact protective services.

At your request, we will give you information on how you may contact protective services for children, adults, or older persons. We will do this confidentially.

You have the right to participate in clinical research when it is appropriate.

Your care provider will discuss this with you when it is appropriate. The institutional review board, a committee that includes people from many parts of this community, monitors all research at BAMC. We will thoroughly explain the proposed research to you and ask your written permission to take part. If you choose not to take part in the research, it will not affect the care that we give you. Participation is completely voluntary.

You have the right to speak to a BAMC patient representative regarding any aspect of your care.

We encourage patients and families to speak directly with ward or clinic personnel if there is a problem; however, if these people cannot solve it, you may contact the patient representative at 916–2330 (clinics) or 916–2200 (inpatient tower).

You have the right to expect that this institution will operate according to a code of ethical behavior.

The command at BAMC is firmly committed to managing this hospital according to the highest traditions of the military and medical professionalism and ethics. In addition, our institutional bioethics committee meets regularly to review ethical topics, including organizational ethics. This committee is available to you and to our employees if a serious ethical dilemma comes up in either patient care or service.

You have a right to receive a personal copy of these patient rights.

Copies of these patient rights are available on any ward and in any clinic at BAMC. If you cannot locate a copy for yourself, ask ward or clinic personnel. If you have any questions or comments regarding patient rights, we encourage you to contact a BAMC patient representative at 916–2330 or 916–2200.

Your Responsibilities as a Patient

You are responsible for maximizing your own healthy behaviors.

You are responsible for taking an active part in decisions about your health care.

You are responsible for providing us with accurate and complete information about your health and your condition.

You are responsible for showing courtesy and respect for other patients, families, hospital staff, and visitors. This includes personal and hospital property.

You are responsible for keeping your scheduled appointments on time and for giving us advance notice if you must cancel or reschedule.

You are responsible for providing us with your current address and means of contact (such as a home phone or cell phone).

You are responsible for providing us with current information regarding any other health insurance coverage you have.

You are responsible for keeping yourself informed of the coverage, options, and policies of the TRICARE plan that you subscribe to as a military beneficiary. This information is available in the TRICARE Service Office (Beneficiary Line: 1–800–406–2832).

Sample Patient Rights and Responsibilities Document (Brooke Army Medical Center, San Antonio, Texas): Spanish Version

Brooke Army Medical Center

Derechos y responsabilidades de los pacientes (al 19 de septiembre de 2.005)

En Brooke Army Medical Center (BAMC) consideramos que el bienestar y seguridad del paciente es nuestra mayor prioridad. *La persona mas importante en este centro médico es usted,* nuestro paciente. Nuestro objetivo es brindarle la major atención médica disponible. Nuestro éxito se verá reflejado en su satisfacción con el tratamiento que recibe. Le damos una gran importancia a sus derechos humanos básicos. Usted tiene derecho a tomar sus proprias decisiones y a saber que sus derechos humanos serán preservados y respetados. La siguiente es una lista de derechos y responsabilidades de los pacientes.

Sus derechos como paciente

Usted tiene el derecho a recibir un tratamiento y servicio respetuoso, considerado y sustentador. Daremos lo mejor de nosotros para brindarle una atención respetuosa y compasiva en todo momento. Haremos todo lo possible para brindarle un ambiente hospitalario seguro. Usted es responsible de mantenerse informado de la cobertura, opciones y políticas del plan TRICARE a que usted suscribe como beneficiario militar. Esta información se encuentra disponible en la Oficina de Servicios de TRICARE (Linea para beneficiarios: 1–800–406–2832).

No discriminaremos para brindarle la atención de la mejor calidad possible en función de: su capacidad de pagar su factura hospitalaria, posición económica, raza, etnia, origin nacional, religión, género, edad, incapacidad física o mental, información genética, orientación sexual o fuente de pago. El acceso a las clínicas ambulatorias es de conformidad con las normas de TRICARE.

Usted tiene el derecho a involucrarse en todos los aspectos de su atención. Nos aseguramos de que sepa que el médico o proveedor de atención es principalmente responsible por su atención. Explicaremos la posición profesional y el rol de las personas que ayudan en su atención. Lo mantendremos totalmente informado de su estado. Le explicaremos claramente todos los tratamientos o procedimientos que propongamos. Nos aseguraremos de que usted participe en el proceso de toma de decisiones sobre su atención. Cuando haya dilemas o diferencias en las decisiones sobre su atención, lo incluiremos a usted para resolvarlas.

Con su permiso, involucraremos a su familia en las decisiones acerca de su atención médica. Solicitaremos su consentimiento por escrito para los procedimientos que implican más que un riesgo mínimo. Respetaremos su derecho a rechazar la atención que aconsejamos. En algunas circunstancias, especialmente para los pacientes en servicio activo, las leyes a reglamentos pueden anular este derecho.

Respetaremos su directiva anticipada con respecto a los limites para la atención que usted desea recibir, de conformidad con la ley de Texas. Respetaremos su orden de no resucitar fuera del hospital en la clínica ambulatoria si se presenta una copia de la directiva y el médico interviniente declara que concide con la directiva. También tiene derecho a indentificar a un tomador de decisiones sustituto para el caso en que usted se vea incapacitado mediante un poder medico.

Tomaremos sus dudas y reclamos con seriedad y trabajaremos duro para solucionarlos. Por lo tanto, estaremos atentos a sus necesidades y pedidos específicos, entendiendo que no deberían interferer con la atención médica para usted y los demás.

Usted tiene derecho a recibir una evaluación y manejo oportuno y apropriado de su dolor. Le preguntaremos sistematicamente si siente dolor. En caso afirmativo, lo evaluaremos y lo ayudaremos a obtener alivio.

Usted tiene derecho a que se respeten sus necesidades personales. Respetaremos la confidencialidad de su información personal en toda la institución y únicamente la divulgaremos de conformidad con las leyes y reglamentos aplicables. Para las personas en servicio activo, puede no ser possible mantener la confidencialidad completa, conforme a los requisitos de informar algunas condiciones y hallazgos. Respetaremos su necesidad de privacidad en las conversaciones, estudios, información compartida y procedimientos. Asimismo, puede soliticar la presencia de un acompanante durante un estudio o procedimiento. Tiene derecho a la divulgación total de la información sobre su salud y a la protección contra la divulgación no autorizada de la información sobre su salud.

Nos comunicaremos con usted en la idioma que pueda comprender. Podemos proporcionar intérpretes y servicios de traducción. Respetaremos su necesidad de sentirse seguro en todas las instalaciones. Los empleados del hospital serán identificables a través de distintivos o credenciales.

Usted tiene derecho a la seguridad física en nuestras instalaciones y nuestro personal de seguridad trabaja las 24 horas del día para garantizarle seguridad.

Usted tiene derecho a su dignidad y sus valores, creencias y preferenicas religiosas, espirituales, culturales y psicosociales. Nuestros proveedores de atención pastoral y espiritual (a menudo llamados capellanes) llevan a cabo visitas diarias a los pacientes y se encuentran a su disposición.

Además, a pedido, coordinan otro apoyo espiritual que usted solicite siempre que no interfiera con su atención médica y la de otras pacientes o el funcionamiento del hospital.

Respetaremos su necesidad de comunicarse con otros, tanto familiars como amigos. Si es clinicamente necesario limitar su comunicación con otros, los mantendremos a usted y su familia informado del motivo. Mientras este internado, lo ayudaremos a realizar conversaciones telefónicas privadas, si lo desea.

Utilizaremos dispositivos de restricción física de tela suave con su monitoreo estricto y frecuente, si usted se encuentra en un estado de confusión tal que corra peligro de lastimarse a si misma o a otros. Quitaremos la restricción en cuanto podamos hacerlo con seguridad.

Usted tiene derecho a estar libre de abuso, negligencia y explotación en casa y en el hospital. Le haremos preguntas sobre estos temas para poder ayudarlo.

Usted tiene derecho a recibir información sobre como contactar servicios de protección. Si la solicita, le brindaremos información sobre como puede contactar servicios de protección y defensora para niños, adultos o ancianos.

Usted tiene derecho a participar en investigaciones clínicas cuando sea apropriado. Su proveedor de atención alanizará esto cuando sea apropriado. La Junta de Revision Institucional, un cómite que incluye a personas de muchas partes de esta comunidad, monitorea todas la investigaciones realizadas en el

BAMC. Le explicaremos detalladamente la investigación propuesta y solicitaremos su autorización escrita para participar. Si decide no participar en lal investigación, esto no afectará la atención que le brindamos. La participación es completamente voluntaria.

Usted tiene derecho a hablar con un representante de pacientes de BAMC con respecto a cualquier aspecto de su atención, incluso para presenter una queja. Alentamos a los pacientes y sus familias a hablar directamente con el personal clinica o de guardia si hay un problema. No obstante, si estas personas no pueden resolvarlo, puede comunicarse con el representante de pacientes al 916–2330 (clínica) o al 916–2200 (torre de pacientes internos).

Usted tiene derecho a esperar que esta institución funcione conforme a un código de comportamiento ético. Usted tiene derecho a estar involucardo en la resolución de dilemas con respecto a su atención, tratamiento y servicios. BAMC esta firmamente comprometido a manejar este hospital conforme a las más elevadas tradiciones de profesionalismo y ética military y médica. Además, nuestro Cómite de Bioetica Institucional se reune con regularidad para revisar temas éticos, incluyendo ética organizacional. Este cómite esta a su disposición y la de nuestros empleados si surge un dilema ético serio en la atención o los servicios de cualquier paciente.

Usted tiene derecho a recibir una copia personal de estos derechos de los pacientes. Las copias de estos derechos y responsabilidades de los pacientes están disponibles en todas las guardias y clínicas de BAMC. Si no puede encontrar una copia, solicítela al personal de guardia o de clínicas.

Si tiene alguna pregunta o comentario con respecto a los derechos o responsabilidades de los pacientes, lo alentamos a que se cominque con un representante de pacientes de BAMC al 916–2330 (clínica) o al 916–2200 (torre de pacientes internos).

Sus Responsabilidades como Paciente

Usted es responsable de maximizar sus propios comportamientos saludables.

Usted es responsable de brindarnos información precisa y completa sobre su salud y su estado.

Usted es responsable de de tomar parte activa en las decisiones sobre la atención de su salud. Usted es responsible de hacer preguntas y seguir las instrucciones de su médico.

Usted es responsable de de mostrar cortesía y respeto hacia los otros pacientes, familiares, personal del hospital y visitas. Esto incluye los bienes del hospital.

Usted es responsable de de ser punctual para sus citas programadas y de avisarnos con anticipación si debe cancelar o reprogramar una cita.

Usted es responsable de brindarnos su domicilio actual y los medios de contacto (tales como telefono particular o celular).

Usted es responsable de de brindarnos información actual sobre cualquier otra cobertura de seguro de salud que posea, y de asegurar que las obligaciones financieras asociadas con su atención se cumplan de manera oportuna.

Sample HIPAA Privacy Notification, English Version

XYZ Rehabilitation Clinic
654 1st Avenue, SW
Majestic, USA 15551
(210) 555-HELP

CLINIC PRIVACY POLICY

Effective date: April 16, 2003

THIS NOTICE INFORMS YOU OF THE PROTECTIONS WE AFFORD TO YOUR PROTECTED HEALTH INFORMATION (PHI). PLEASE READ IT CAREFULLY.

Purpose: HIPAA, the Health Insurance Portability and Accountability Act of 1996, is a federal law addressing privacy and the protection of protected health information (PHI). This law gives you significant new rights as to how your PHI is used. HIPAA provides for penalties for misuse of PHI. As required by HIPAA, this notice explains how we are obliged to maintain the privacy of your PHI and how we are permitted by law to use and communicate it.

Maintenance of records: We use and communicate your PHI for the following reasons: treatment, reimbursement, and administrative medical operations.

- **Treatment** includes medical services delivered by professionals, for example, an evaluation by a doctor or nurse.
- **Reimbursement** includes activities required for reimbursement for services, including, among other things, confirming insurance coverage,

sending bills and collection, and utilization review, for example, sending off a bill for services to your company for payment.

- **Administrative medical operations** include the business of managing the clinic, including, among other things, improving the quality of services, conducting audits, and client services, for example, patient satisfaction surveys.

We also are permitted to create and distribute anonymous medical information by removing all references to PHI.

All of the employees of this clinic may see your records, as needed. We use sign-in and sign-out logs containing the names of our patients in the waiting room, and we telephone patients to confirm appointments. We place your folder in a plastic in-box (with your name hidden) in the hallway in front of your treatment room.

When making photocopies of your records, we have your folder in our sight at all times until we file it away with other folders. The medical records area is limited to employees only. When we send your PHI by fax, we ensure to the maximum extent possible that the receiving fax is secure.

All other uses of your PHI require your written authorization, including sharing your PHI with family members or others. You have the right to revoke any authorization in writing, and we have the legal duty to comply with such a revocation, except to the extent that we have used your information in reliance on your previous authorization or as required by law.

The right of patients to see, copy, and amend their medical records: To take advantage of these rights, please present your request in writing to the clinic privacy officer (discussed later here). You have the right to see your medical records. We will try to give you access as quickly as possible, depending on our load. Within 1 week of your request, you may see your records in one of our offices, with the assistance of one of our employees. You have the right to make copies of your records. We have the right to charge for those copies. You may also request that the privacy officer honor special limitations on the uses and communications of your PHI. We are not obliged to comply with such requests. If we agree, we have to comply with the request until you advise us in writing otherwise. You have the right to receive a copy of this notice, which we offer to you on your first visit. This notice, which is subject to change, is posted prominently in our waiting area.

Privacy Officer: The privacy officer for the clinic is _____ _____, RN. Please speak with this employee about any question or complaint that you may have about your PHI. You may make special requests concerning your PHI.

Correspondence with the patient: We will send correspondence to the address that you have given us, but you have the right to ask that we send correspondence to a different address.

Complaints: If you feel that your PHI has not been treated with privacy, you may communicate this concern to the clinic privacy officer. You also have the right to communicate any problem to the Secretary of Health and Human Services (a division of the federal government) without being worried about retaliation by this clinic. We ask, however, that you first discuss and try to resolve any problem with our privacy officer. Thanks, and welcome to XYZ Clinic!

Sample HIPAA Privacy Notification, Spanish Version

Clinica XYZ de Rehabilitación
654 1st Avenue, SW
Majestic, USA 15551
(210) 555-HELP

NORMA DE PRIVACIDAD DE LA CLÍNICA

Fecho efectivo: 16 de abril de 2.003

ESTA NOTICIA LE INFORMA SOBRE LAS PROTECCIONES QUE TOMAMOS CON SU INFORMACIÓN MÉDICA PROTEGIDA. HAZ FAVOR DE LEERLO CON CUIDADO.

Intento: HIPAA, el Health Insurance Portability and Accountability Act of 1996, es una ley federal que trata con la privacidad y protección de información médica protegida (IMP). Esta ley le da a usted, el paciente, derechos significantes nuevos sobre como se utiliza su IMP. HIPAA provee por penas por el mal uso de IMP. Como es requisito por HIPAA, esta norma explica como estamos obligado de mantener la privacidad de IMP y como estamos permitido usar y comunicar su IMP.

Mantenamiento de los documentos: Utilizamos y comunicamos su IMP por las razones siguientes: el tratamiento, el pago y las operaciones administrativas médicas.

- **Tratamiento** incluye servicios medicales entregados por profesionales. Ejemplo: evaluación por un médico o enfermera.

- **Pago** incluye actividades requisitas para el reembolso de servicios, incluyendo, entre otras cosas, confirmar los seguros, mandar facturas y colecionar, y analisis de utilización. Ejemplo: mandando una factura a su compañia de seguro para pagar por servicios.

- **Operaciones administrativas médicas** incluyen el negocio de administrar la clínica, incluyendo, entre otras, el mejoramiento de la calidad de servicios, hacer auditorias, y servicio de clientes. Ejemplo: encuestas de satisfacción.

También podemos hacer y distribuir información médica anónima por quitar todas referencias a la IMP.

Todos los empleados de esta clínica pueden ver sus documentos, si necesitan verlos. Usamos planillas de firmar al entrar y salir, anunciamos los nombres de nuestros pacientes en la sala de espera, y llamamos a pacientes para recordarles de sus citas. Pondremos su carpeta de documentos en un caja plastica (con nombre escondido) en el pasillo de su cuarto de tratamiento.

Al hacer copias de sus documentos, tendremos la carpeta en nuestra vista hasta que lo guardamos con las otras carpetas. La área en que guardamos las carpetas está limitada a sólo los empleados. Cuando mandamos sus documentos por fax, nos aseguramos lo más possible que el fax a donde lo mandamos esté seguro.

Todos otros usos de su IMP requiere su autorización escrito, incluyendo el compartamiento de su IMP con familiares u otras personas. Tiene el derecho de revocar su autorización en escrito, y tenemos la responsabilidad de cumplir con tal revocación, excepto al punto que ya hemos usado la información dependiente de su autorización anterior, o cuando tenemos que comunicar información por ley.

El derecho de los pacientes a ver, copiar y enmendar sus documentos médicos: Para ejecutar estes derechos, por favor presente su petición en escrito al oficial de la privacidad (vea abajo). Usted tiene el derecho de ver sus documentos médicos. Trataremos de rápidamente darle aceso, dependiente en lo ocupado que estemos. Entre una semana después de su solicitud, podrá ver los documentos en una sala de esta oficina, con la asistencia de un empleado. Tendrá el derecho de hacer copias. Tenemos el derecho de cobrar por las copias. También puede pedir al oficial de la privacidad peticiones especiales sobre los usos y comunicaciones de su IMP. No tenemos que cumplir con estas peticiones. Si estamos de acuerdo, tenemos que seguir con la petición hasta que usted acuerde en escrito de quitarla. Tiene el derecho de tener una copia de esta noticia, que le ofrecemos en su primera visita a la clínica. Esta noticia, que se puede cambiar, esta puesto prominentemente en la sala de recepción.

Oficial de la Privacidad: El oficial de la privacidad de la clinica es
_____ _____, RN. Por favor, hable con este empleado sobre cualquiera pregunta o queja que tenga sobre su IMP. Puede pedirle cosas en especial sobre su IMP.

Correspondencia al paciente: Mandaremos cartas a la dirección que usted nos ha dado, pero tiene el derecho de pedir que las mandemos a otra dirección.

Quejas: Si usted piensa que su IMP no ha sido tratado con privacidad, usted puede comunicar este problema al oficial de la privacidad de la clínica. También tiene el derecho de comunicar cualquier problema al Secretario de Health and Human Services (division del gobierno federal) sin preocupaciones de retaliación de esta clínica. Le rogamos que hables primeramente con el oficial de la privacidad para resolver problemas. ¡Gracias y bienvenido a la clínica XYZ!

Sample Resume: Spot the Actual and Potential Errors (10 or More)

John Paul Doe

4410 Main Street
San Antonio, Texas 78001
Age: 18

Home: 210-555-1314
DOB: Dec. 19, 1978
Marital Status: Single

OBJECTIVE: To obtane a position as a health services clinical manager. I am limited (because I am single father) to employment within south central Texas.

EXPERIENCE: *2004–present* San Alexis Medical Clinic
111 S. Main, SATX 78110 210-555-1212

Medical office administrator: Duties included supervising staff of two. Salary: $15,500 annually. Reason for leaving: Seeking better benefits package with paid continuing education.

2002–2004 Tom Thumb Middle School
Justice ISD Wonderful Town, TX 210-555-1243

6–12 Health teacher. Reason for leaving: I hurt my back lifting boxes at work.

2001 Willis Lake Middle School 210-555-1666

Student Teaching

EDUCATION: *1997–2001* Southcentral Texas State University
Santa Vida, TX

B.S., Health/Business. *Ipsa Contra Ipsa* Faternity.

REFERENCES: Jim Doe. Manager, Acme Science Shop, Confine, TX. Relation: uncle. Worked at his store in summers 1995–6.

Father Xavier McLeod. St. Mary Magdalene Church, San Antonio, TX. Parish priest.

Sample Resume
With Errors Corrected

John Paul Doe

4410 Main Street
San Antonio, Texas 78001

Home: 210-555-1314
Cell: 210-555-8911
Email: jpd@YourSite.com

OBJECTIVE: To use my best skills and practices as a clinical manager to impart optimal quality care to patients and clients and their significant others and to continue my professional, educational and personal development

EXPERIENCE: *2004–present* San Alexis Medical Clinic
111 S. Main, San Antonio,
Texas 78110   210-555-1212

Medical Office Administrator: Reorganized outpatient files into color-coded folders for easy retrieval. Led successful JCAHO survey, Aug. 2005. Employee of the year, 2005.

2002–2004 Tom Thumb Middle School
Justice ISD   Wonderful Town, TX   210-555-1243

6–12 Health Teacher: Initiated student-led district health science fair. New Teacher Excellence Award 2003.

2001   Wood Lake Middle School   210-555-1666

Student Teaching: 6–12 Regular and Honors Health

EDUCATION: *1997–2001* Southcentral Texas State University
Santa Vida, TX

Bachelor of Science Degree, Dual Health
Education/Business Major
Minor: Exercise and Sports Science
Dean's List
6–12 Health Education Certification, 2001

AVOCATIONS: International travel (I have lived in Germany and Spain); conversational in Spanish; play guitar and piano.

REFERENCES: Available upon request

Sample Cover Letter

May 31, 2006

Jim Johnson
Director of Human Resources
ABC Medical Center
1112 East Main Street
San Antonio, Texas 78111

Dear Mr. Johnson,

I am writing to follow up with you after our telephone conversation of May 23, 2006. I called you because I am seeking a position as an outpatient clinical manager. You asked me to send you my resume, which I have attached.

I have had an opportunity to research ABC Medical Center and find it to be a superb and highly respected urban medical center, serving area disadvantaged patient populations. I believe that my education and background, enthusiasm, knowledge of Spanish, and strong drive to serve disadvantaged and all other patient populations in the San Antonio area make me a very competitive candidate for a position as an outpatient clinical manager.

Your advertisement in last Sunday's *Express News* lists available openings for clinical managers in dermatology, outpatient surgery, and physical medicine and rehabilitation. I am interested in applying for any of the three positions. I am particularly interested in the challenging environment of outpatient surgery.

Thank you for speaking with me and for your attention to my resume. I look forward to hearing from you and hopefully being invited to interview at ABC.

Respectfully,

Reginald P. Hausenfus III

Index